Thinking About Thinking

Orlando N. Acosta

Thinking About Thinking

Copyright © 2016 by Orlando N. Acosta. All rights reserved.

Contents

Preface   5

Figures   7

1   The Nervous System for Humans an Elementary Description.   9
    1.1 Human's nervous system   9
    1.2 The CNS   11
    1.3 The PNS   14
    1.4 Neurotransmitters   19
    1.5 Neurotransmitters receptors   20
    1.6 Neurons discovery and classification   21
    1.7 Neurons outer membrane and structure   23

2   Neuron Cells   28
    2.1 Excitable cells   28
    2.2 Sensory neurons   30
    2.3 Motor neurons   31
    2.4 Interneurons   31
    2.5 The plasma membrane   32
    2.6 Nissl Bodies   34
    2.7 Mitochondria   34
    2.8 Endoplasmic Reticulum   37
    2.9 Golgi Apparatus   38
    2.10 Vesicles   39
    2.11 Lysosomes   40
    2.12 Nucleus   41
    2.13 Dendrites and Axons   42

3   Neuron's Resting Potential   44
    3.1 Resting potential   44
    3.2 Action potential generation   46
    3.3 The refractory period   49

4	**Glial Cells**	**51**
	4.1 Introduction	51
	4.2 Astrocytes	52
	4.3 Oligodendrocytes	58
	4.4 Ependymal cells	58
5	**Thinking About Thinking**	**60**
	5.1 Questions	60
	5.2 Humans thinking process	61
	5.3 Thinking restrictions	62
	5.4 It is a human world	67
6	**Thinking Patterns**	**69**
	6.1 Introduction	69
	6.2 The electric and magnetic fields	71
	6.3 Quantum electrodynamics	73
	6.4 Vision and the human eyes	76
	6.5 The retina	80
	6.6 Sensory patterns	84
	6.7 Alzheimer's brain disease	85
	6.8 Neural networks and artificial intelligence	91

Appendix 1 Action potential illustration   95

Preface

The human nervous system and especially the brain presents a real conundrum to scientist and physicians alike. They know where everything is and how it looks, but they don't know how it works. And nowhere this is more evident than in the brain. Actually, wise men and researches are starting to lose hope of understanding the riddle. They know that nothing would really change in the next few decades, and perhaps centuries. Philosophers will argue that it will never happen.

In chapter 5, I bring into focus the limitations of the human mind and the restrictions inherent in our reasoning process. For a long time, researchers have been looking for the "thinking cell or organelle" that would explain how we think and memorize; they had found nothing. In section 5.1, I argue that the mind produces theories, ideas, and concepts through reasoning and reasoning implicitly conveys restriction. Hence, man cannot make rationalizations without restriction.

In chapter 6, I introduced the concept of thinking patterns. Although, the present day knowledge about thinking patterns is almost zero. We know that each of these patterns contains billions of neurons, and even more of the many types of glial cells, and Schwann cells, and that blood capillaries provide blood to the patterns.

The interactions between all these components is largely unknown. But what is completely unknown is how we memorize information, and how we reason about it.

In sections 6.4, 6.5 and 6.6 I present my ideas about human vision and how it works. And stated that the electromagnetic field of the reflected light mimics, exactly and instantaneously the shape, size, and color of the object that reflected the light. **There is not other plausible explanation.** The confirmation of this statement could have important consequences in physics. In Section 6-6 I put forward the idea that the information contained in the reflected light is directly correlated to the shape of the electric field equipotential surfaces in the sensed pattern.

To make the book more readable, I repeated in Chapter 2 some information already covered in Chapter 1. Although I have not attempted to give specific credit at each point, I used material from the internet as a source of data and information. I draw up figures 1-2, 6-8 and Appendix I, all the other figures were copied from the internet.

Orlando N. Acosta, MSEE

04-17-2017

Figures in Thinking about Thinking

Fig. 1-1 Cerebral Cortex

Fig. 1-1A Parts of the human brain

Fig. 1-1B Brain's regions and what they do and control.
Fig. 1-2 Illustration of typical sensory neurons

Fir. 2-1 Neuron structure

Fig. 2-2 Mitochondria and their structure by Kelvisong; modified by Sowlos

Fig. 2-3 Different types of endocytosis.

Fig. 4-1 Four types of Glial Cells in the Central Nervous System. Ependymal, Astrocytes, Microglial and Oligodendrocytes.
Fig. 4-2 Types of glial cells

Fig.4-3 Glial cells of the CNN.

Fig. 4-4 Glial cells of the PNS.

Fig. 4-5 Illustration shows Ependymal and Neuroglial Cells.

Fig. 6-1 Electromagnetic wave illustration.

Fig. 6-2 Cross section of the human eye
Fig.6-3 Retina's structure.
Fig. 6-4 Illustration shows the distribution of cones and rods in the fovea area.
Fig. 6-5 Response of cones to light spectrum

Fig. 6-6 Population of photoreceptors in the most sensitive part of the retina.
Fig. 6-7 Brain area activated when observing an object.
Fig. 6-8 Illustration of Amyloid Beta creation.
Fig. 6-9 Brain comparison.
Appendix 1 Action potential illustration

Chapter 1

The Humans' Nervous System, an Elementary Description.

If it is alive, it thinks! Therefore, all animals, cells and organelles think, there is no other way to explain their performance.

1.1 Human's nervous system.

The nervous system of humans, is the culmination of a very long evolutionary process that began with the first signs of life on the planet earth. Although we can recognize some shortcomings in this compact and neatly packed system, among them: bad actuators and long computation time. It is also true that we cannot design or built anything as efficient as the human nervous system. The adaptation of the species to the earth environment and the built-in requirement that to survive and reproduce it was necessary to perform better than anything around has proven to be a better design tool than the human's brain. Human reasoning is no match for the evolution process. Humans are still in the classification phase of our analysis of the nervous system. Here are the results of this effort.

- A live human brain is soft and fatty looking; it weighs 3 pounds approximately or 2.5 % of the average human being weight (120lb).
- It has a total surface area (including the area hidden by the folds) of 324 square inches and a volume of 85 cubic inches.
- It contains an estimated 200 billion neurons and more than 3,000 billion glial cells or **neuroglia**, meaning nerve glue.

Glial cells (discovered in 1891 by Santiago Ramon y Cajal) do not communicate using neurotransmitters and until recently the general consensus was that they don't participate in the thinking, sensing, motoring and controlling processes taking place within the brain. Glial cells are smaller but more abundant, at least by a factor of ten, than neurons. In fact, they are a major component of the brain tissue, with more than one half its weight. It has been known for many years (since early in the 20th century) that glial cells provide structural and nutritional support to neighboring neurons. Furthermore, they regulate the amount of fluid surrounding neurons and help to break down some of the neurotransmitters used by them. Glial cells, found in the *brain and the spinal cord,* are classified in two main branch **Macroglia** and **Microglia.** Macroglia cells could be astrocytes, oligodendrocytes, and glioblasts.

Astrocytes are star shaped cells and are characterized by featuring many projecting long arms or processes often ending in button or plate like

expansions. There are two types of astrocytes:
- **Protoplasmic.** Found in the gray matter and their processes are thick and symmetrically spaced.
- **Fibrous.** Found in the white matter with thin and asymmetrical spaced processes.

Oligodendrocytes: They are small cells without processes, and unlike astrocytes contain many organelles in their bodies as well as many microtubules. They generate the myelin layer that surrounds, protect and insulate the neuron's axons. In a similar way, outside the central nervous system, the Schwann cells (first cousins of the oligodendrocytes) perform the same mounting function of the peripheral nerves that connects the brain and the spinal cord with glands, muscles, and sensory organs of the human body.

Glioblasts: They are stem cells, which could evolve into glial cells.

1.2 The CNS

The nervous system is composed of the Peripheral Nervous System (PNS) and the Central Nervous System (CNS). The central nervous system consists of the brain and the spinal cord. The *brain,* see Figs. 1-1, 1-1A, and 1-1B interacts with the external environment and the human body. Actually, it dedicates most of its volume and controlling power to process and to act on the sensory information it receives from 12 pairs of cranial nerves and from the spinal cord. The *spinal cord* transmits sensory information from the PNS to the brain, and transmits motor commands from the brain to a diverse assembly of muscles and glands. The brain as well as the spinal cord are wrapped and protected by three layers of connective tissue called the meninges. They are called: Dura Mater, Arachnoid, and Pia Mater. The outermost layer, the Dura Mater, cushions the CNS against impacts with the bones of the cranium and vertebrae. The brain depends for its survival on an uninterrupted supply of blood; which provides not only glucose and oxygen, but also is the source of cerebral-spinal fluid, which contains considerable less protein than most extracellular fluid elsewhere in the human body. The cerebral-spinal fluid runs through the entire central nervous system before is reabsorbed into the blood stream. It fills the four brain cavities and circulates continuously around the brain perimeter between the arachnoid and the Pia matter meninges and through the cerebrum-spinal canal of the spinal cord. The cerebrum-spinal fluid is produced inside the brain ventricles by the choroid plexuses, which are the hairy formations lining parts of some of the ventricles. Both the brain and the spinal cord contain white matter and gray matter. The white matter consists of bundles of myelin coated neuron's axons. The gray matter consists of accumulations of neuron's bodies and dendrites bunched together forming solid masses. The surface of the brain consists of gray matter and the inner side consists of white matter. In the spinal cord the surface is white and the inside is gray.

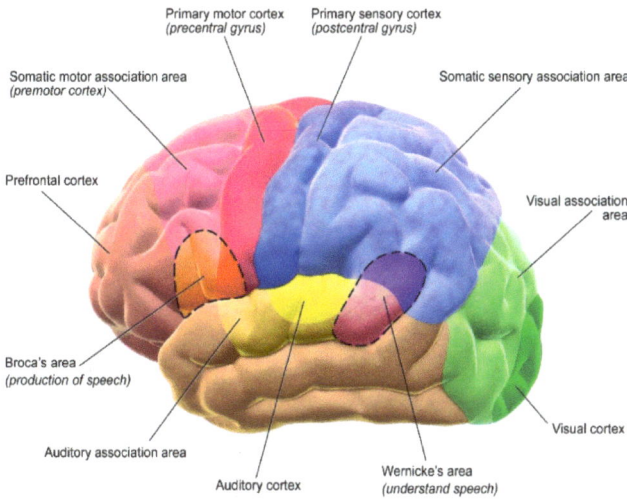

Figure 1-1 Cerebral Cortex.
Blausen.com staff (2014). "Medical gallery of Blausen Medical 2014". *WikiJournal of Medicine* **1** (2). DOI:10.15347/wjm/2014.010. ISSN 2002-4436. - Own work

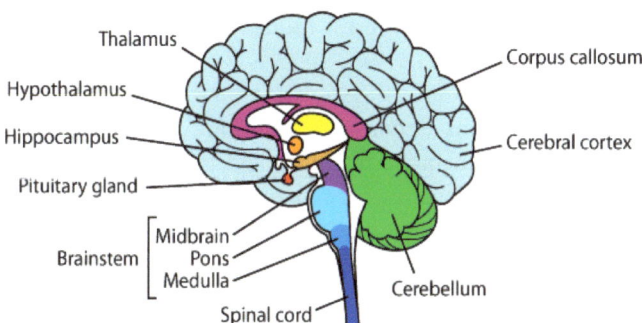

Figure 1-1A Parts of the human brain.

By Brett Szymik. "A Nervous Journey."
ASU - Ask A Biologist. 5 May 2011.
http://askabiologist.asu.edu/parts-of-the
brain.

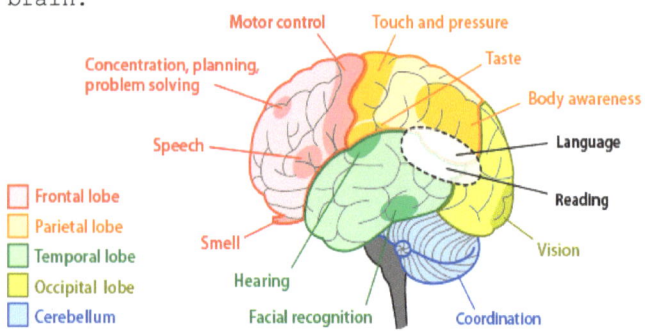

Figure 1-1B Brain's regions and what they do and control.
By Brett Szymik. "A Nervous Journey."
ASU - Ask A Biologist. 9 May 2011.
http://askabiologist.asu.edu/brain-regions.

1.3 The PNS

The peripheral Nervous System is formed by sensory and "motor" neurons functioning outside of the central nervous system. Typical neurons of the PNS are illustrated in Fig. 1-2. **A cluster of neuron's bodies is called a ganglion. Many neuron's axons bundled together is called a nerve.**

The peripheral Nervous System covers the entire human body. Its neurons divide and subdivide forming a tree that reaches the most recondite parts of the body. It consists of 12 pairs of cranial nerves residents in the periphery of the brain and 31 pairs of nerves emanating from the spinal cord. Sensory neurons transmit stimuli information from the stimulus receptors to the CNS. Motor neurons transmit action commands from the CNS to the effectors: muscles, glands, and organs.

The PNS has two main branches: The sensory-somatic nervous system (SSNS) and the autonomic nervous system (ANS). The SSNS interacts with the external environment. Our awareness of the external environment and our motor reactions to deal with it are handled by the SSNS. The ANS controls the internal body environment.

The SSNS consists of the 31pair of nerves emanating from the spinal cord and some of the 12 pairs of cranial nerves. One nerve from each pair serves one side of the body, the other nerve serves the other side of the body. All the 31 pairs emanating from the spinal cord are mixed, because they contain sensory and motor neurons. However, the cranial nerves, could be entirely sensory, like the olfactory nerves (first pair), or entirely motion producing, like the oculomotor nerves (third pair), or mixed like the fifth pair, the trigeminal nerves.

The ANS consists of sensory and motor neurons. They carry operating information and commands from the CNS, mainly from the hypothalamus, the medulla oblongata, and the spinal cord to most of the organs of the human body. This amazing system tracks the performance of the human organs, and induce in anyone of them whatever correction or change is necessary to maintain our body working, as well as it can. And do this automatically, without a need for us to think about it. The operation of the ANS is easier to understand if it is separated into two parts, each acting in opposition to the other. The part that controls the highs is called the sympathetic nervous system, and the part that controls the lows is called the parasympathetic nervous system.

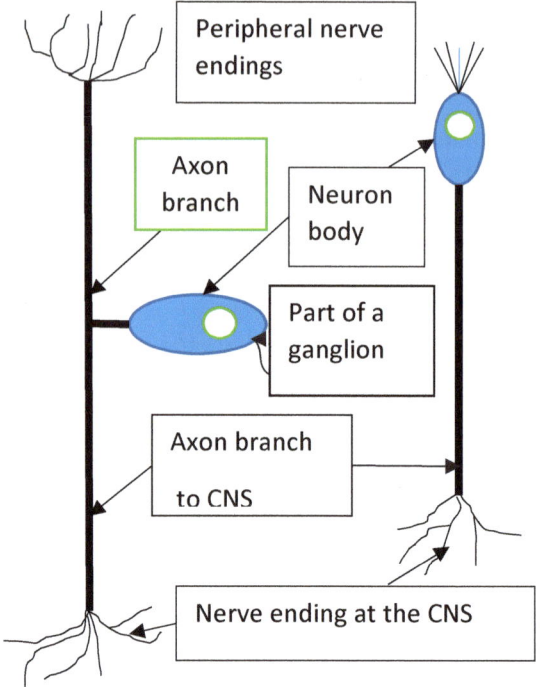

Figure 1-2 Illustration of typical sensory neurons

The Sympathetic Nervous System. In this system, a nerve impulse or command does not go directly to its destination. It goes first to a sympathetic ganglion (mass of specialized neurons or nerve cells) and from there it switches to another neuron before arriving to the target organ. Most of the nerves of this system originate in the thoracic and lumbar regions, the middle section of the spinal cord. The preganglionic motor neurons of the sympathetic nervous system have short axons to connect the spinal cord with sympathetic ganglions located very close to the spinal cord. The postganglionic neurons, in contrast, have long axons to connect the ganglions with the target organs, glands, or muscles.

There are two vertical chains of sympathetic ganglions symmetrically arranged on either side of the spinal cord. Once a nerve impulse (action potential), transmitted via a motor neuron (preganglionic neuron) of the sympathetic nervous system arrives to a ganglion of the ganglionic chain, it can proceed in four different ways:

1. Some of them synapse (connect) right there with another neuron (postganglionic) which in turns delivers the action potential to the target organ, gland or muscle.

2. Keep going up or down the ganglionic chain until it encounters the preferred ganglion where it connects with a postganglionic neuron and keeps going to the target. How the human brain selects the appropriate ganglion? No one really knows.

3. Exit the first ganglion via a nerve cord on its way to the solar plexus, the largest ganglion of the ANS, situated in the abdominal cavity, behind the stomach, just below the diaphragm, where it synapses with postganglionic neurons leading to the target organ.

4. Some preganglionic neuron passes right through the solar plexus in its way to the adrenal medulla where it synapses with special sympathetic postganglionic neurons that are part of the secretory portion of the adrenal medulla.

The actions (excitation or inhibition) induced by the sympathetic system could be felt by all the cells of the human body. A single neuron could synapse with specialized neurons in the secretory part of the adrenal medulla and induce the release of adrenaline into the blood stream, ensuring that all the cells of the human body are exposed to the stimulation originated in the sympathetic portion of the autonomic nervous system. This clearly is a survival mechanism, it prepares the body for emergencies, one for instance, could be: fight or run for your life.

<u>The Parasympathetic Nervous System.</u>
From the medulla oblongata, located within the hindbrain (Which includes: Pons, medulla oblongata, and cerebellum.) at the tip of the spinal cord, emanates the main nerve of the parasympathetic nervous system and possibly the single most important nerve in the body. It is the tenth pair, one of the twelve pairs of cranial nerves. This numbering system was introduced in the second century AD by Galen, the legendary Greek physician. This all important nerve is called the **Vagus** nerve and is the longest of the cranial nerves. It runs from the medulla oblongata through the face and thorax to the splenic flexure of the colon. It is a mixed nerve with sensory and motor neurons, and it branches into many organs and muscles. It reaches the heart, lungs, stomach, kidneys, liver, and intestines. This wandering nerve regulates breathing, heartbeat, digestion, and controls the movements of many muscles of the mouth. It helps to control the speech and facilitates breathing by keeping the larynx open.

Others preganglionic nerves of the parasympathetic system originate in the brain and some others originate in the lower tip of the spinal cord. The ganglions of the parasympathetic system are located close the target organs. So, the preganglionic neurons have long axons and the postganglionic neurons have short axons.

The parasympathetic system returns the function of the body's organs to normal after they have been

inhibited by the actions of the sympathetic system. So the parasympathetic system could induce the following:
- Decreases the blood pressure
- Increases the flow of blood to the skin and viscera
- Decreases the heartbeat
- Constricts the pupils of the eyes
- Constricts the bronchi
- Contracts the bladder
- Stimulates peristalsis and secretions in the gastrointestinal tract
- Stimulates the production of saliva
- Stimulates the secretion of bile in the liver.

1.4 Neurotransmitters.

Some neuron transmits nerve impulses across the synaptic cleft by discharging molecules of specific chemicals, called neurotransmitters, into the synaptic cleft. The human central nervous system operates by means of a multitude of neurotransmitters. There is a family of neurotransmitters, called peptide neurotransmitters, in which more than 50 of them have been identified. They transmit sensory and emotional responses, like: pleasure, pain, hunger, thirst and sex drive. Why so many? No one knows. Maybe is to separate the instructions emanating from the CNS.

All the preganglionic neurons of the autonomic nervous system, transmit action potentials to the postganglionic neurons by means of the neurotransmitter acetylcholine; which is also the neurotransmitter used by motor neurons in the sensory somatic nervous system. So, it is safe to say that acetylcholine is the neurotransmitter that the nervous system releases to activate muscles. And that is also used by the autonomic nervous system, in both the sympathetic and in the parasympathetic nervous systems. Furthermore, acetylcholine is the chemical that the brain uses not as a neurotransmitter, but to modify the way that other parts of the brain process information.

The neurotransmitter secreted by most of the postganglionic neurons of the sympathetic nervous system into the target organ is Norepinephrine (also called noradrenaline), in some excitatory synapses the neurotransmitter consists of a combination of norepinephrine and Adenosine triphosphate (ATP) molecules. But, the neurotransmitter secreted by most of the postganglionic neurons of the parasympathetic nervous system into the target organ is also acetylcholine. Some of the postganglionic neurons of the parasympathetic system in the gastrointestinal tract use nitrous oxide (a soluble gas) instead of acetylcholine to transmit their nerve impulses. Nitric oxide neurotransmitters are not encapsulated inside vesicles.

Some other neurotransmitters are: Dopamine, Serotonin, Endorphins, Norepinephrine, GABA (Main inhibitory neurotransmitter in the brain,) Glutamate (Main excitatory neurotransmitter in the brain). We don't know very well which neurotransmitters are used by the interneurons of the CNS (Brain and spinal cord).

1.5 Neurotransmitter receptors.

Once a neurotransmitter is discharged into the extracellular fluid at the synaptic cleft it interacts with a postsynaptic receptor at the postsynaptic neuron, although in some cases the receptor is located at the presynaptic neuron itself. Some specific chemicals could mimic the action of some specific neurotransmitters, these chemicals are called **agonists.** They bind to receptors and could generate postsynaptic potentials. For instance, **nicotine** is agonist to acetylcholine; it binds to acetylcholine receptors. The exact synaptic action depends on the neurotransmitter receptor combination. Acetylcholine neurotransmitters and nicotinic receptors are the combination used by all the *preganglionic* or somatic motor neurons of the CNS. The *postganglionic* neurons of the sympathetic nervous system use norepinephrine (or noradrenaline) as neurotransmitter in combination with adrenergic (adrenaline like) receptors. These adrenergic receptors are located in such vital organs as: heart, lungs, kidneys, etc. **There is an entire family of drugs called Beta-blockers (antagonist to norepinephrine) whose main function is to reduce the blood pressure, cardiac arrhythmia, and chest pain. Beta-blockers compete with the neurotransmitters (norepinephrine) for the receptor sites at the heart muscle, in this way they control the heartbeat rate by interfering with the action of the norepinephrine.** Another example is the "Curare" a drug which is antagonistic to acetylcholine neurotransmitter. The Curare binds to acetylcholine receptors at nerve muscles and blocks the muscular action. In the parasympathetic nervous system, the postganglionic neurons that use acetylcholine as Neuro transmitter depends of muscarinic receptors.

1.6 Neurons discovery and classification

In 1865 Otto Dieters, of Bonn, Germany, published the first realistic drawing of a neuron. Santiago Ramon y Cajal (1906 Nobel prize winner for medicine) the famous Spanish histologist proved that the nervous system consists of a web of independent neurons.

Neurons are excitable cells specialized to receive and transmit electrochemical impulses called action potentials or nerve impulses. Neurons are independent structures, not connected to each other. **However, their most remarkable quality is that they are capable of working in groups forming thinking patterns.** Neurons patterns not only could memorize information, but also are capable of producing rational thinking, of learning very complex task, and of creating or inferring new ideas or concepts based on what we already know. A great collection of neurons forms our brain, but a collection of patterns (networks) forms our mind. We know nothing about neurons and glia cell networks, except that we must conclude that they exist. There isn't another way to explain the accomplishments of the human mind. Indeed, they are responsible for everything produced by the human intellect.

Our science is based on structures that are formed by other more elementary structures or particles. So we have atoms formed from electrons, protons and neutrons. And molecules formed by atoms organized by chemical bonds. In contrast, neuron-glia cell networks are just neurons-glia cells working together to accomplish complicated tasks. And unlike the case with atoms and molecules we discover the elementary particles of the neuron-glia cell networks before we could prove the network's existence.

Neurons are classified into three types: sensory, motor, and interneurons. Sensory neurons are those that connect stimulus receptors (vision, sound, odor, taste, and touch) or sensory cells with the central nervous system (the brain, and the spinal cord). The bodies of sensory neurons synapsing with interneurons in the spinal cord form dense masses called dorsal ganglions.

Motor neurons are those that transmit impulses or action potentials from the central nervous system to the muscles and glands that implement the commands emanating from the CNS.

Interneuron is a type that includes a conglomerate of many different kinds of neurons with great diversity of structural and functional specialties. **These are the thinking neurons.** The **brain** has about 200 billion of them (also, there are interneurons in the spinal cord), this is an estimated number which is constantly growing. It is estimated that the average number of synapses of each interneuron is 1000 (another big guess).

Of all the neurons, interneurons are the ones we know less about. This is due to the many difficulties researchers experience when trying to study interneurons in actual working conditions, without harming the human submitted to the experiment. Besides, interneurons poor performance is not considered to be a disease, although the impact of this flaw could have far reaching consequences.

Interneurons connect only with other neurons and unlike motor or sensory neurons their axons stay within a specific location within the brain or spinal cord. Besides being part of the thinking patterns (networks); they are intermediary signal processors. **But what makes this type of neurons unique is that they can communicate among them without using neurotransmitters. Some pairs of interneurons are, in fact, electrically coupled.**

1.7 Neurons outer membrane and structure

Neurons, like all the other cells in the human body, have an outer membrane, a nucleus and a body containing a gel like, clear fluid called the cytoplasm. However, neurons specific features make them very different from all other cells. Neurons don't reproduce, therefor they are the oldest and longest cells in the human body. Some neurons are never replaced when they die, but many last for the entire life of a person. In contrast, most of the human body cells, with the exception of heart and skeletal muscle cells, multiply continuously during a lifetime.

Neuron's structure evolved (we believe) as a result of the functions they most perform. There are minor structural differences between some neurons of the peripheral system and those of the central nervous system, but in general terms a neuron consists of:

- The plasma membrane which surrounds the cell body.
- The cell body which is filled with a fluid called cytoplasm, which contains several specialized structures or organelles.
- The nucleus.
- Dendrites.
- Axon hillock, axon, and axon terminals.

The plasma membrane is a double layered (lipid bilayer), fluid like envelope that support, protects and contribute to the neuron's maintenance. The plasma membrane is impermeable to:

- Charged particles such as: K^+, Na^+, Ca^{++}, and Cl^-
- Small hydrophilic molecules like glucose.
- Macromolecules like proteins and RNA

However, there is a constant passage of ions and molecules from the extracellular fluid to the cytoplasm inside the neuron and the other way around. The transport of these particles through the *impermeable* membrane is accomplished as follows:

By *facilitated diffusion*. Transmembrane proteins (membrane embedded proteins) create water filled pores which some ions and small hydrophilic molecules use to penetrate the plasma membrane by diffusion.

By *active transport*. Some other ions and small molecules depend on transporters to cross the plasma membrane. These transporters are specialized membrane embedded proteins which use the energy released by ATP molecules to push charged particles against the repulsion of an electrical field or against the concentration gradient for no charged particles. Membrane embedded proteins play a multitude of roles in neurons: Besides transporting molecules and ions in and out of neurons, they are essential in receptor recognition and in neuron to neuron (synapse) communication.

By *endocytosis*. Macromolecules suspended in the extracellular fluid use endocytosis to cross the membrane. This is the process that neurons use to engulf large proteins and Ribonucleic acid (RNA), a macromolecule made up of nucleotides. During the engulfing process an endosome, a membrane-bound vesicle, is formed around the engulfed particles. Eventually, the particles contained in the vesicle are released into the cytosol. See Fig. 2-4.

Inside the neuron's body, which is no wider than 100 microns (0.1 millimeters) and could be as tiny as 4 microns wide, there are several structures immersed in the cytoplasm, see Figure 2-1, they are:

1. **Nissl Bodies** or groups of ribosomes that are essential in the synthesis of protein. A neuron contains hundreds of thousands of ribosomes, the number depends on the amount of protein

produced by the neuron. Some ribosomes are contained in the cell cytoplasm others are contained inside mitochondria. The ones inside mitochondria are smaller (0.02 microns) than the ones resident in the cell cytoplasm.
2. **Endoplasmic Reticulum (ER)** which is a very intricate structure formed by membranes, tubules, and vesicles. It retains, transports and purified materials within the cytoplasm. There are two kinds of ERs: the smooth ER (SER) and the rough ER (RER).
3. **Golgi Apparatus.** All the proteins produced by the RER must travel to the Golgi Apparatus where they are chemically treated and packed for traveling to their final destination inside or outside the neuron.
4. **Vesicles** are transport vehicles used by all human cells including neurons. There are two types of vesicles: Transport Vesicles, which are the ones that move materials between organelles of the same neuron. And Secretory Vesicles, which are used to ship materials out of the neuron.
5. **Lysosomes** are the neuron's trash collector. They have spherical bodies enclosed by a single membrane. Their main function is to expel some materials from the neuron, to transform others into forms that could be digested and assimilated by the neuron, and to do all these without threatening the neuron itself. The exocytosis of lysosomes is the mechanism that neurons use to repair wounds in their plasma membrane.
6. **The nucleus** storage and manage the use of the neuron's genetic material. The nucleus is

contained inside a very complex nuclear envelope that consists of a double lipid bilayer membrane. A lamina lying beneath the membrane provides structural strength to the nuclear envelope. Inside the nucleus, suspended in the nucleoplasm, are dense strand of nucleoprotein fibers holding the neuron's genetic material.
7. **Dendrites and Axons** are extensions emanating from the cell body. Dendrites bring signals to the cell body and axons carry signals away from the cell body. In general, neurons have many dendrites but only one axon. Axons are covered by a smooth myelin jacket; dendrites don't have a myelin layer. Axons don't contain ribosomes, dendrites do. Dendrites branch off near the cell body, axons branch off far away from the cell body. The part of the cell body that connects with the axon is called **axon hillock**. The cell body and dendrites are covered by thousands of hair like extensions of the cytoplasm, the hillock has none.

The active transport, through the neuron's membrane, in opposite directions, of sodium ions and potassium ions carried out by the ATPase pump produces the following results:

Outside the neuron, at rest, the concentration of sodium ions (Na+) is ten times greater than inside.

Inside the neuron, at rest: the concentration of potassium ions (K$^+$) is twenty times greater than outside. Meanwhile, the ionic concentrations of chloride (Cl$^-$) and calcium ions (Ca^{++}) are kept at higher levels outside the neuron. However, inside the neuron, in some membrane bound pockets, the concentration of calcium ions (Ca^{++}) could also be very high. At rest, the potential inside the neuron with reference to the immediate outside settles at the value of -70 millivolts.

Chapter 2

Neuron Cells.

2.1 Excitable cells

In 1865 Otto Dieters, of Bonn, Germany, published the first realistic drawing of a neuron. Santiago Ramon y Cajal (1906 Nobel prize winner for medicine) the famous Spanish histologist proved that the nervous system consists of a web of independent neurons. Based on this solid foundation, neurons were recognized as the main component of the nervous system and that they were the key to understand how our brain works.

Neurons are excitable cells specialized to receive and transmit electrochemical impulses called action potentials or nerve impulses. Neurons are independent structures, not connected to each other. However, their most remarkable quality is that *they are capable of working in groups forming thinking patterns. Neurons patterns not only could memorize information, but also are capable of producing rational thinking, of learning very complex task, and of creating or inferring new ideas or concepts based on what we already know.* A very large group of many billions of neurons and glial cells constitutes our brain, but an assemblage of neurons and glial cell patterns (networks?) make our mind. We know nothing about neurons and glia cell patterns, except that we must conclude that they exist. There isn't another way to explain the accomplishments of the human mind. Indeed, they are responsible for everything produced by the human intellect.

Our science is based on structures that are formed by other more elementary structures or particles. So we have atoms formed from electrons, protons and neutrons. And molecules formed by atoms organized by chemical bonds. In contrast, neuron-glia cells patterns are just neurons-glia cells working together to accomplish complicated tasks. And unlike the case with atoms and molecules we discover the neuron's organelles (elementary particles) before we could prove the patterns existence. For many years researches had been looking inside neuron cells trying to find the thinking organelle (particle). Their motto should be: **if it is alive it thinks! Therefore, all cells and organelles think.** There is no other way to explain their performance.

Neurons are classified into three types: sensory, motor, and interneurons.

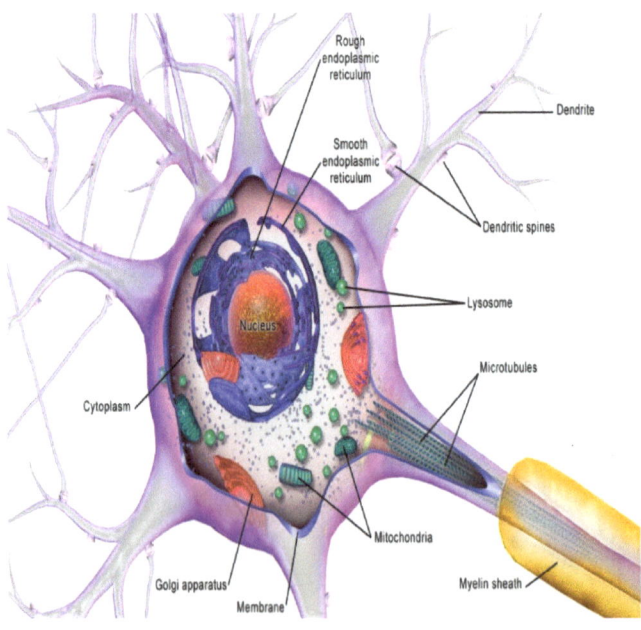

Figure 2-1 Neuron structure
By Bruce Blaus-Own work, (CCBY-SA4.0),
https://commons.wikimedia.org/W/index.php?curid=46621398

2.2 Sensory neurons
Sensory neurons are those that connect stimulus receptors (vision, sound, odor, taste, and touch) with the central nervous system (brain, and the spinal cord). The bodies of sensory neurons synapsing with interneurons in the spinal cord form dense masses called dorsal ganglions. See Fig. 1-2.

2.3 Motor neurons
Motor neurons are those that transmit impulses or action potentials from the central nervous system to the muscles and glands that implement the commands emanating from the CNS.

Inside the neuron's body, which is no wider than 100 microns (0.1 millimeters) and could be as tiny as 4 microns wide, there are several structures immersed in the cytoplasm, see Fig. 2-1, they are: Nissl Bodies, Mitochondria, Golgi Apparatus, Endoplasmic Reticulum, and Nucleus.

2.4 Interneurons
This type of neurons includes a conglomerate of many different kinds of neurons with great diversity of structural and functional specialties. These are the "thinking" neurons. The brain has about 200 billion of them, this is an estimated number which is constantly

growing. This number does not include the interneurons in the spinal cord. It is estimated that the average number of synapses of each interneuron is 1000 (another big guess). Of all the neurons, interneurons are the ones we know less about. This is due to the many difficulties researchers experience when trying to study interneurons in actual working conditions, without harming the human submitted to the experiment. Besides, interneurons poor performance is not considered to be a disease, although the impact of this flaw could have far reaching consequences.

Interneurons connect only with other neurons and unlike motor or sensory neurons their axons stay within their specific location in the brain or spinal cord. Besides being part of the thinking patterns (networks); they could be intermediary signal processors. **But what makes this type of neurons unique is that they can communicate among them without using neurotransmitters. Some pairs of interneurons are, in fact, electrically coupled.**

Neurons, like all the other cells in the human body have an outer membrane, a body that contains a nucleus and other organelles; all immersed in a gel-like, clear fluid called the cytoplasm. However, neurons have some specific characteristics that make them very different from all other cells. Neurons don't reproduce, therefore they are the oldest and longest cells in the human body. Some neurons are never replaced when they die, and many last for the entire life of a person. In contrast, most of the human body cells, with the exception of heart and skeletal muscle cells, multiply continuously during a lifetime.

2.5 The plasma membrane

This membrane consists of two layers of phospholipids (fatty acids) with embedded proteins protruding from their surfaces. Each layer has a hydrophilic (like water) surface and a hydrophobic (it doesn't like water) surface. The membrane assembly resembles a sandwich, in which the water loving side of one layer faces the intracellular space and the water loving side of the other layer faces the cell's cytoplasm. The membrane is a fluid, like-envelope that enclose the cytoplasm and performs many different tasks:
1. Accumulates cell nutrients, rejects damaging particles
2. Its encrusted proteins catalyze some enzymatic chemical reactions.
3. It is a control barrier that regulates the ionic flow **in** and **out** of the cell body.

The plasma membrane is:
- **Selectively** permeable to some ions such as: K^+, Na^+, Ca^{++}, and Cl^-. The degree of permeability is not equal for these ions. The membrane is more permeable to potassium, chlorine comes next, and sodium is the least permeable of them.
- **Impermeable** to small hydrophilic molecules like glucose.
- **Impermeable** to some macromolecules like proteins and RNA.

However, there is a constant traffic, in both directions, of ions and molecules, between the extracellular fluid and the cytoplasm inside the neuron. To reach equilibrium, ions prefer to move from high to low concentrations. Any difference in ionic concentration density across the membrane is called **concentration gradient**. If there is a difference between the same sign ionic concentration densities across the membrane, there is a voltage difference across the membrane, and therefore an electrical field exists across the membrane. Transporting these ionic particles through the "impermeable" membrane is accomplished as follows:

1. *Facilitated diffusion*. The transmembrane proteins embedded in the membrane create water filled pores. Some ions and small hydrophilic molecules use these water filled pores to penetrate the impermeable membrane by diffusion.
2. *Active transport*. Some ions and small molecules depend on transporters to cross the plasma membrane. These transporters are **specialized membrane embedded proteins** which use the energy released by adenosine triphosphate (ATP) molecules to push charged particles against the repulsion of the electrical field or against the concentration gradient for non-charged particles. ***Membrane embedded proteins play a multitude of roles in neurons: Besides transporting molecules and ions, in and out of neurons, they are essential in receptor recognition and in neuron to neuron communication (synapse).***
3. Endocytosis is the process neurons use to engulf large proteins and Ribonucleic acid (RNA.) During the engulfing process an **endosome**, which is a membrane-bound vesicle, is formed around the engulfed particle. Eventually, the particle contained in the vesicle is released into the cytosol. See Fig. 2-3. Succinctly, macromolecules suspended in the extracellular fluid are transported across the neuron membrane by endocytosis.

2.6 Nissl Bodies

They consist of **groups of ribosomes** that are essential in the synthesis of proteins. A neuron contains hundreds of thousands of ribosomes, the number depends on the amount of protein produced by the neuron. Some ribosomes are contained in the cell cytoplasm others are contained inside mitochondria. Those inside mitochondria are smaller (0.02 microns) than those residing in the neuron cytoplasm.

2.7 Mitochondria

These organelles have a very complicated "bacterial-like genesis." The quantity of mitochondria contained in the cytoplasm of a neuron vary according with the cell's needs. Mitochondria are the neuron's source of energy, because they have the enzymes required to transform glucose and oxygen into adenosine triphosphate (ATP). Neurons use the chemical energy stored in ATP to do most of their biochemical reactions, for instance the ATPase pump consists of specialized membrane embedded proteins which use the energy released by ATP molecules to push charged particles against the repulsion of an electrical field or against the concentration gradient for non-charged particles. A mitochondrion **is the holder of its own DNA, independent of the neuron's genome, which is contained in its nucleus.** Some cells do not have mitochondria, others, like liver cells have a lot of them, around 2000 per cell. Mitochondria length varies in the range of about 0.75 -3 microns and besides filling the neuron's energy needs, they perform many other tasks, for instance: they control the neurons life cycle (growth, cellular differentiation, and death.) The structure of a mitochondrion is organized by compartments, where, in each of them, unique and specialized functions are carried out. These compartments are: the outer membrane, the intermembranes space, the inner membrane, the cristae and the matrix. See Fig. 2.2. The outer membrane is 0.75 microns thick and it contains a large number of porins (membrane proteins) which form channels that make the outer membrane permeable to small molecules. Actually, the small molecule concentration in the intermembrane space is the same as in the neuron's cytosol. However, the protein composition of the intermembrane space is not the same than the protein composition of the neuron's cytosol, because some large molecules could bind to a protein in the outer membrane and get a ride across the outer membrane into the neuron's cytosol. The outer membrane of a mitochondrion contains many enzymes that carry out many essential structural and chemical tasks. The free ribosomes contained inside a mitochondrion are essential for its protein production. The inner membrane is impermeable to all sizes of molecules, because it does not contain porins. In fact, to enter or exit the matrix which is the space inside the inner membrane, see figure 2-2, molecules as well as ions require special membrane transporters. As shows in figure 2-2 the inner membrane is not linear, but wavy, this increases the membrane surface area; in fact, the area of the inner membrane is five times larger than the area of the outer membrane. And as shown in figure 2-2 the undulations or folds of the inner membrane are called **cristae**. Figure 2-2 shows the cristae surfaces are studded with F particles. Inside the matrix there is plethora of hundreds of enzymes, mitochondrial ribosomes and several copies of the mitochondrial DNA genome. The inner membrane contains ATP synthase, which is a key ingredient for the production of ATP.

Some cells have a very high quantity of mitochondria because they use a lot of energy.

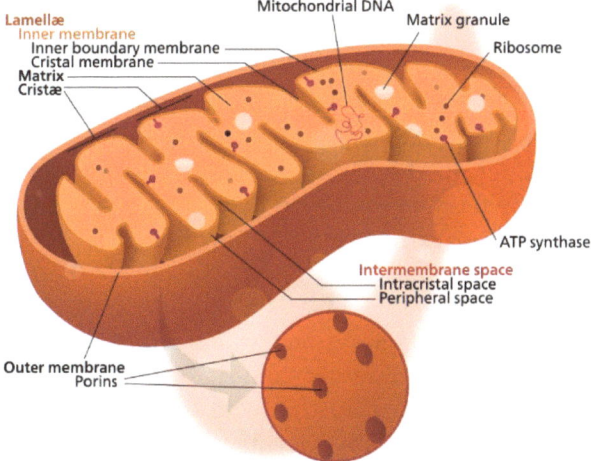

Figure 2-2 Mitochondria and their structure by Kelvisong; modified by Sowlos - Own work, based on: Mitochondrion mini.svg, (CC BY-SA 3.0), https://commons.wikimedia.org/w/index.php?curid=27731882

The separation between mitochondria and the endoplasmic reticulum could be very small, in the range of 10 – 25 nanometers. The membrane like organelle that connects the mitochondria with the endoplasmic reticulum is called MAM (Mitochondria Associated Membrane). The MAM size is about 20 percent of the outer membrane size.

2.8 Endoplasmic Reticulum

The Endoplasmic Reticulum (ER) is a very intricate structure formed by membranes, tubules, and vesicles. It retains, transports and purifies materials within the cytoplasm. See Fig. 2-1. There are two kinds of ERs: the smooth ER (SER) and the rough ER (RER). The SER is formed by a labyrinth of membranes and tubules and it does not have ribosomes encrusted on its surface and therefore is considered smooth. The SER participates in the detoxification of poisons and in the synthesis of lipids (fats, waxes, cholesterol, steroids, etc.) The neuron's smooth endoplasmic reticulum is not large compared to the SER of some specialized cells of the liver and kidney. Another function of the SER is the isolation of calcium ions, it prevents their movement inside the cytosol.

The rough endoplasmic reticulum (RER) consists of a series of membranes, standing in a formation of parallel sheets connected by the tubules. The surface of these membranes is encrusted with protein synthesizing ribosomes. The RER is located near the nucleus and serve as a bridge between the nuclear envelope and the Golgi Apparatus. The main function of the RER is the synthesis of proteins, including neurotransmitters. *All the proteins produced by the RER must travel to the Golgi Apparatus where they are chemically treated and packed for their final destination, inside or outside the neuron.*

2.9 Golgi Apparatus

The Golgi Apparatus (GA) is formed by a stack of 4 to 6 compartments of flattened sacs, or cisterns each containing specific processing enzymes. In these sacks the protein molecules synthesized in the Endoplasmic Reticulum are modified, encapsulated inside vesicles, and send to their final destination. The compartment where proteins enter the GA is the cisface and the compartment where they exit is the transface. Proteins are sequentially modified by the enzymes as they move throughout the cisface, the midfaces, and the transface of the GA. The movement is carried out by transport vesicles. Proteins to be used outside the neuron are placed in the proper secretory vesicles by a precise sorting process, which occurs in the final compartment, of the transface of the GA. Proteins inside this final compartment are recognized by chemical flags.

2.10 Vesicles

Vehicles are used by all human cells, including neurons. There are two types of vesicles: *Transport Vesicles*, which are the ones that move materials between organelles of the same neuron. *Secretory Vesicles,* are used to ship materials out of the neuron. Transport vesicles are created in the membrane of the shipping organelle. See figure 2-3. A portion of the membrane of the shipping organelle, close to the target particle, changes from straight to **loop-like** and surrounds the target particle. After completing the particle engulfing, the squeezed part of the organelle's membrane pinches off, and becomes the membrane of the transport vesicle itself. Vesicles move toward their destination following the grain of the cell cytoskeleton. When a vesicle reaches its destination, it fuses with the membrane of the receiving organelle and discharge its content.

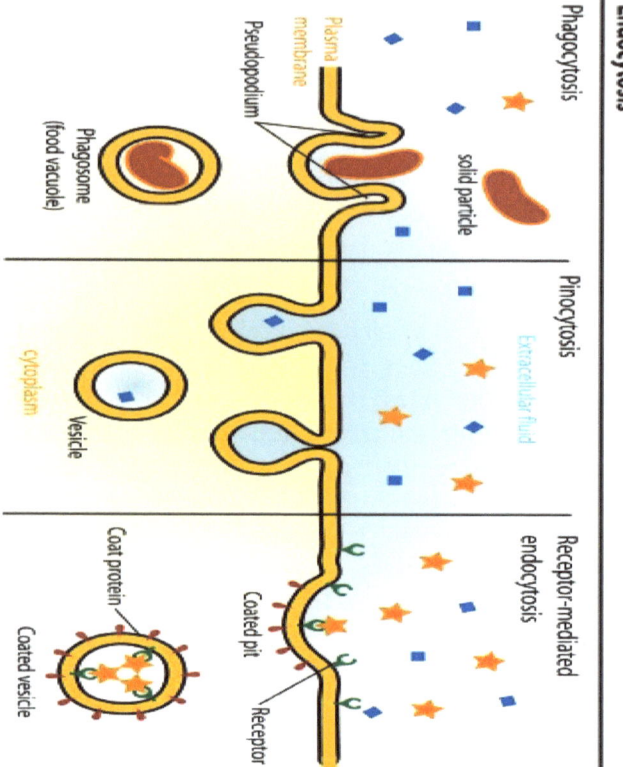

Figure 2-3 Different types of endocytosis.
The copyright holder of this work released it into the **public domain**.

2.11 Lysosomes

Lysosomes are the neuron's trash collector. They have spherical bodies enclosed by a single membrane. Their main function is **to expel** some materials from the neuron, **to transform** others into forms that could be digested and assimilated by the neuron, and to do all these without threatening the neuron itself. The exocytosis of lysosomes is the mechanism that neurons use to repair wounds in their plasma membrane. **Lysosomes are created in the Golgi apparatus** and travel to the neuron surface where they become attached to the plasma membrane. Lysosomes contain forty different kinds of hydrolytic enzymes (acid hydrolases). This doesn't mean that a particular lysosome would contain the forty types of hydrolytic enzymes. These enzymes are used to break down or transform all sorts of macromolecules before they could be assimilated or excreted. The hydrolytic enzymes are produced in the RER, modified at the Golgi Apparatus, and shipped inside vesicles to the lysosomes. Materials to be digested by a neuron are first deposited within lysosomes. For instance, dead mitochondria, food molecules, bacteria....

Lysosomes remove macromolecules by excreting them inside secretory vesicles. And transform sugars, amino acids, and nucleotides into new forms that could be used by the neuron. To do their work the 40 types of enzymes exist in different concentrations, and all of them are acid hydrolases with an optimal working environment with a pH of 5. Because the neuron's cytosol is mildly basic (pH of about 7.2), the lysosomes processing enzymes can't work within this environment and therefore they don't present a risk to the neuron itself in case they leak into the cytoplasm.

2.12 Nucleus

The *nucleus* storage and manage the neuron's genetic material. The nucleus is contained inside a very complex nuclear envelope that consists of a double lipid bilayer membrane. A lamina lying beneath the membrane provides structural strength to the nuclear envelope. Inside the nucleus, suspended in the nucleoplasm, are the dense strand of nucleoprotein fibers holding the neuron's genetic material. The nuclear envelope completely surrounds the nucleoplasm and acts as a barrier to: ions such as K^+, Na^+, Ca^{++}, $Cl-$ and to small water soluble molecules like glucose. Clusters of proteins attached to the membrane surface of the nuclear envelop form a basket like apparatus (the nuclear pore complex). This basket facilitates the flow of RNA (Ribose Nuclei Acid) and proteins in and out of the nucleus.

The nucleus has chromosomes with the required genetic information for development of the host neuron and for the synthesis of the required proteins for neuron's maintenance and survival. The nucleus encloses a dense eye shaped structure called the nucleolus. It produces RNA subunits and ribosomes. These materials pass throughout the nuclear membrane into the neuron's cytoplasm where the ribosomes can actually convert genetic information into proteins.

2.13 Dendrites and Axons

Dendrites and axons are extensions emanating from the cell body. The consensus is that dendrites bring signals to the cell body and axons carry signals away from the cell body. In general, neurons have many dendrites but only one axon. Axons are covered by a smooth myelin jacket; dendrites don't have a myelin layer. Axons don't contain ribosomes, dendrites do. Dendrites branches are close to the cell body. Axons branch-off far away from the cell body. The part of the cell body that connects with the axon is called axon **hillock**. The cell body and dendrites are covered by thousands of hair like extensions of the cytoplasm, the hillock has none.

The neuron body and the nucleus don't participate in the transmission of nerve impulses. Their primary function is to keep the neuron alive, in working conditions. However, the axon *hillock* is where the initiation of the nerve impulse or action potential usually occurs. No all the nerve impulses are initiated in the axon hillock; some are generated in dendrites. If the ***total*** stimulation resulting from the addition (to be confirmed) of all the triggering signals is greater than a threshold value established at the axon hillock, then the neuron fires and transmit the nerve impulse, via the axon and dendrites to other neurons, cell muscles, or cell glands. The nerve impulse strength is independent of the number of synapses; it reaches **each** synaptic gap with the same intensity it has at the axon hillock or dendrite.

The axon grows out of the neuron's body, it is a long, tubular like, thin extension of the cell cytoplasm. It could be several feet long and only a few microns in diameter. Besides of conducting nerve impulses the axon transport cellular materials by way of many microtubules (approximately 0.025 microns in diameter) running inside the axon. However, electron microscope photos show than rather than microtubules the neurons transport system consists of strands of hyper-phosphrylated tau proteins layout in parallel tracks resembling, in a very minute scale, a railroad system. It could well be that the **"tracks"** transport not only neuron's nutrients, but also data (not necessary in electrical form), and perhaps, tracks are the key for us to understand "micro-reasoning".

Most axons are contained in a fatty sheath formed by the expanded membrane of Schwann cells. These cells are located at regular intervals along the axon and their expanded membranes wrapped around the axon forms a myelin jacket that insulates and covers the axon. There is a gap in between adjoining Schwann cells, these gaps are called nodes of **Ranvier**. In these gaps the axon is bare; without the protection of the insulating jacket.

Chapter 3

Neuron's Resting Potential

3.1 Resting potential.

The separation of charges (cations/anions) across the cytoplasm membrane of all cells, excitable or not, produces an electric field and a difference in the electrical potential across the cell's membrane. In steady state condition, the interior of the cell is negative with respect to the exterior. The potential difference across the cytoplasm membrane, when the cell is in a steady state condition is called the ***resting potential***. In this state the cell is considered to be at rest, although working hard to keep living.

When a **neuron** is not excited, at steady state condition (at rest), its resting potential is -70 millivolts. If the neuron's cytoplasm membrane were permeable to charged particles, any difference in ionic concentration (for any specific ion) between the interior and the exterior of the neuron would eventually balance out. But the neuron's membrane is very selective. Actually, it has channels dedicated to control the flow of each type of ion. The resting potential is the result of the following activity:

1. When the neuron is at rest some ions of potassium (K^+), sodium (Na^+) and chloride (Cl^-) can cross the cytoplasm membrane. They tend to migrate to the side of the plasma membrane that have an electrical potential opposite to its electrical charge. Potassium is the one that crosses more readily, sodium and chloride ions have more difficulty. However, negatively charged protein molecules inside the neuron are not able to cross the plasma membrane due to their size, charge or structure.

2. The main factor that contributes to establish and maintain the value of the resting potential is the sodium/potassium pump, also called the ATPase pump, which provides the necessary energy to push out of the neuron, against the electro-chemical potential gradient, three sodium ions ($3Na^+$) for every two potassium ions ($2K^+$) it moves in. Enzyme: Na^+ / K^+ pump or ATPase pump or sodium-potassium adenosine triphosphate pump.

This enzyme is found in the plasma membrane of all animal cells, including, of course, in all neurons of the human brain. The neuron's cytoplasm membrane contains many adenosine triphosphate (ATP) molecules, and they consume up to two thirds of each neuron total energy consumption. In this process the ATP molecule is

converted by hydrolysis into ADP (Adenosine diphosphate) plus inorganic phosphate plus energy. This reversible process, is used by cells in all forms of life.
Symbolically:
ATP + H2O ----> ADP + Pi + Energy
This process is an active transport of a fixed number of molecules. For each ATP molecule that is hydrolyzed, 3 sodium ions are transported out of the neuron and 2 potassium ions are transported into the neuron.

As a result of the activities described above in 1 and 2, the potential inside the neuron with reference to the immediate outside settles at the value of -70 millivolts.

The active transport, in opposite directions, of **sodium out** and **potassium in** through the neuron's membrane carried out by the ATPase pump produces the following results:
- At rest, outside the neuron: the concentration of sodium ions (Na^+) is ten times greater than inside.
- At rest, inside the neuron: the concentration of potassium ions (K^+) is twenty times greater than outside.

Meanwhile, the ionic concentrations of chloride (Cl^-) and calcium (Ca^{++}) ions are kept at higher levels **outside** the neuron. Furthermore, **inside** the neuron, in some membrane bound pockets, the concentration of calcium ions (Ca^{++}) could also be very high.

3.2 Action potential generation.

When a stimulus, in the form of a voltage spike, reaches a neuron, that is resting it causes the opening of hundreds of voltage controlled *sodium channels* at the neuron's membrane. The sodium ions dwelling outside the neuron's membrane are double motivated to penetrate the membrane. Because the concentration of sodium ions (Na⁺) is ten times greater outside than inside, and the neuron's inside potential is -70 millivolts with respect to the outside. The positive charge of the sodium ions drives the neuron inside potential up toward the plus side with reference to the outside. When the inside potential reaches **-55** millivolts the neuron fires an action potential. As soon as the sodium channels open up an avalanche of sodium ions occurs, and in the fraction of a millisecond (0.5 milliseconds) that the sodium channels remain open several thousands (7000) of sodium ions move to the neuron's inside. The **minus 55** millivolt is a precise threshold level, no nerve impulse will be fired if the potential inside the neuron doesn't reach this critical level. In the presence of a stimulus (or the resultant of many simultaneous stimulus), the neuron either fires a full size action potential or doesn't fire one. For a specific neuron the strength of the action potential is always the same. Furthermore, the action potential strength is independent of the number of synapses; It reaches each synaptic gap with the same intensity it has at the origin, *the axon hillock or dendrite*. The increase of the inside potential ends when the sodium channels close up, but the inside potential doesn't stay there at the tip of the spike, with a value of **+30 millivolts approximately**, for any significant amount of time. Because at this precise moment, when the neuron inside potential is about +30 millivolts with reference to the outside, voltage controlled <u>potassium</u> channels open up at the neuron's membrane and many thousands of potassium cations (K⁺) rush **out** of the neuron. The loss of positive charges drives the neuron inside potential down toward the resting potential of *minus 70 millivolts*, but usually, it goes beyond this value (undershoot) and becomes even more negative, because some potassium channels remains open longer than they should. Finally, one millisecond after the peak (approximately) the neuron's potential reaches the bottom (in the order of minus 77 millivolts). Then, the potential inside the neuron starts to recover and increases toward the -70 millivolts value. The neuron's potential increases slowly and ends at the minus 70 millivolt level, with the help of some leaving chlorine ions, when all the potassium and sodium channels reach their steady state condition. The refractory period is in the order of 1.5 to 2 milliseconds.

The sudden increase of the difference in potential across a specific neuron's membrane is the natural response of the neuron to a set of inputs (as many as several thousand of them) arriving at the neuron by means of the synaptic action with other neurons. The inputs could arrive simultaneously or within a very brief interval of time, less than one millisecond. Although some neurons are capable of integrating inputs (to be confirmed) arriving within a larger interval of time. Some of these synapses are excitatory (tend to increase the neuron's inside potential) and others are inhibitory (tend to decrease the neuron's inside potential).

An action potential would be fired, if the integration of all the excitatory inputs arriving (at different spots of the membrane) within one millisecond minus the integration of all the inhibitory inputs arriving (at different spots of the membrane) within the same one millisecond is larger than the threshold level of -55 millivolts. The evaluation whether to fire or not to fire is made at the *axon hillock*, See Fig. 2-1, perhaps this is why the membrane is bare at this location. There are not synapses (hairs) protruding from the cytoplasm membrane in the area of the axon hillock. Once a neuron fires an action potential it shows, with equal strength, at all (not only at the axon terminals) the synapses of that neuron. A great number of these synapses will in turn induce additional action potentials in several thousand other neurons, and so on. It is, indeed, an exponentially growing activation of neurons. The resulting synapsing action produced by the propagation of many thousands action potentials proceeds toward the intended **target** and must also inform the CNS that the action is proceeding along the right path. No one knows where the propagation stops or how many neurons are affected, but there must be a mechanism in our brain to limit and direct all these activities.

3.3 The refractory period.

Normally, a neuron cannot generate a new action potential while is in the middle of one, it needs to wait until it recovers and the -70 mv resting potential is again established. The refractory period lasts from the peak of the spike to the end of the recovery time, or about 1.5 milliseconds or larger. See appendix 1. The recovery time ends when all the potassium channels are closed and the neuron's membrane resting potential is again established. The illustration depicted in Appendix 1 shows that the refractory period is in fact longer, that it keeps going after all the potassium gates are closed, because the neuron's inside negative potential is still smaller (larger in magnitude) than the required minus 70 millivolts. In fact, it looks like the neuron *realize (?)* that the best way to return its inside potential to minus 70 millivolts is by letting out enough negative electrical charges until the inside of the neuron reaches the steady state potential of -70 mV. This is why some Cl^-

ions leave the neuron during the tail end of the recovery period.

The voltage spike period is the time from stimulus arrival to complete recovery, and in general, is about two milliseconds long. This means that the neuron is capable of firing an action potential every 2 milliseconds or at the rate of 500 action potential per second.

Symbolically: $T = 2/1000$ seconds $\quad f = 1/T = 1000/2 = 500$ action potential per second

If a strong stimulus, stronger than require to initiate an action potential, arrives while the neuron is **recovering**, the neuron could fire an action potential without waiting for arriving at the resting potential first. This period of time is called: **Relative Refractory Period.** But, there is a period of time, when the inside potential of the neuron is *falling* beyond -70 millivolts, in which it is impossible to restart the voltage spike. This period of time is called:

Absolute Refractory Period. Appendix 1 illustrates the refractory periods. The duration of the stimulus, its shape and peak voltage value will affect the duration, shape, and peak voltage of the action potential. In general, If the stimuli are not equal, then the action potentials will be different. However, if the stimuli are all equal; then the existence of a brain "clock" is possible.

Chapter 4
Glial Cells

4.1 Introduction

Glial cells are, the more numerous component of the central nervous system, they support and protect neurons, the main component of the nervous system. Also, glial cells maintain the stability of the central nervous system. The different types, by function, of glial cells in the central nervous system are: **astrocytes, oligodendrocytes, ependymal, and microglia.** See Figs. 4-1, 4-2, and 4-3 The types of glial cells in the peripheral nervous system are: **Schwann, satellite, and enteric glial**. See Figs. 4-3 and Fig. 4-4. It is a complicated world, very compact, in which everyone does what it is supposed to do.

The glial cells obvious functions are:

- To stabilize and maintain neurons in place
- To supply nutrients and oxygen to neurons
- To remove dead neurons.

4.2 Astrocytes

Of all glial cell types in the central nervous system, **Astrocytes** are the type with the largest number of cells. Astrocytes are star shaped because they have many branches radiating in all directions, many of them terminate in flat looking expansions that could attach to blood vessels or other cells, see Fig. 4.3. Two astrocyte types are recognized:

1. Protoplasmic astrocytes, which are found in the gray matter. They have thick symmetrical branches.

2. Fibrous astrocytes, which are found in the white matter. They have thin asymmetrical branches.

Astrocytes are not electrically excitable, but they are very important in the development and physiology of the central nervous system. Here are some of the tasks that astrocytes perform: support the metabolism of neurons, help in the differentiation of neurons, and regulate the local concentration density of ions and neurotransmitters in the extracellular space. Astrocytes also play a role in the control of local blood flow. However, astrocytes are still considered passive cells with no participation in the collection and processing of the information provided by the sense organs to the brain. It could be, that what is really missing or incomplete is our knowledge. Astrocytes communicate with each other by means of electrical synapses, which are much faster than chemical synapses and where the electrical continuity across the narrow gap between pre and post synaptic terminals is established by the flow of ions which in general is bidirectional. However, in some electrical junction the ions can only flow in one direction. These are the so called rectifying junctions. The brain uses this type of junction for nerve firing synchronization. Astrocytes could also use second messengers to bridge the electrical gap junctions between them. Like Inositol Triphosphate (IP3) which diffuse from one astrocyte to another and then binds to the endoplasmic reticulum where it liberates stored Ca^{++} ions by opening ligand gated ion channels and letting the calcium ions out into the cytosol. The liberated calcium ions might increase the production and release of IP3, which would create a calcium wave that quickly spreads from astrocyte to astrocyte. The branches (processes) of astrocytes can move, retract and extend, and therefore they could arrange or modified the extracellular space. Which would transform the geometry of the extracellular space by changing the available space and the clearance between cells that belong to the same pattern. They also regulate the concentration densities of ions and neurotransmitters in the pattern, by removing excess potassium ions and by reusing some surplus neurotransmitters often expelled by neurons from their synaptic cleft. These actions would change the flow of neurotransmitter in the extracellular space. Which means that astrocytes participate in controlling the entire operation of a pattern, and thereby could also participate in the control of muscles and organs.

Likewise, astrocytes could change the coverage of neuronal chemical synapses, which is another way of affecting the pattern internal flow of ions and neurotransmitter and controlling the pattern signal output. Besides, controlling the extracellular concentration, density of potassium ions, astrocytes use glutamate *transporters* to remove glutamate from some chemical synaptic clefts and shut down the operation of some chemical synapses. Glutamate is a very abundant neurotransmitter and both glial cells and neurons use it for communication purposes. It is believed that glutamate account for 90% of the synaptic connections in the brain.

Astrocytes require chemical energy for four general types of tasks: to drive metabolic reactions that would not occur automatically, to transport needed substances across membranes, to move muscles and to communicate with the other atrocities. The required energy is provided by carbohydrates and fat molecules which are then converted into ATP. The ATP molecules deliver the energy to specific places inside astrocytes where the energy is required.

Astrocytes are not electrically excitable instead their communicating work is based on free Ca^{++} ion concentration density changes in their cytosol. The point to point free Ca^{++} concentration variations in the cytosol might be used for communication purposes in a specific astrocyte or from astrocytes to astrocytes, or from astrocytes to neurons. In the last few years the existence of bidirectional communication between astrocytes and neurons has been documented. It does exist, and it makes sense, because they usually are extremely close, separated only by a few microns. Zooming out, the brain looks like a solid mass, like many other organs in the human body do. Why then to assume that the brain cells live independent lives, if they live so close to each other in the brain.

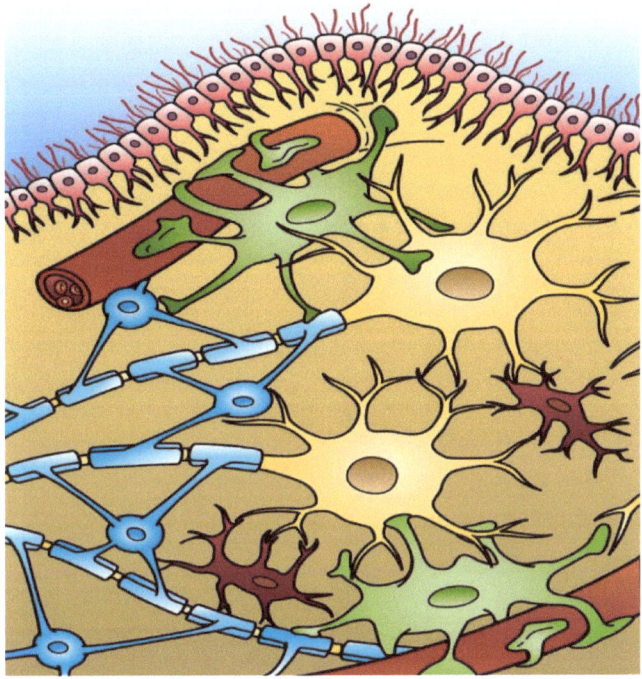

Figure 4-1 Four types of Glial Cells in the Central Nervous System. Ependymal, Astrocytes, Microglial and Oligodendrocytes. Artwork by Holly Fischer [CC BY 3.0

(http://creativecommons.org/licenses/by/3.0)] via Wikimedia Commons.

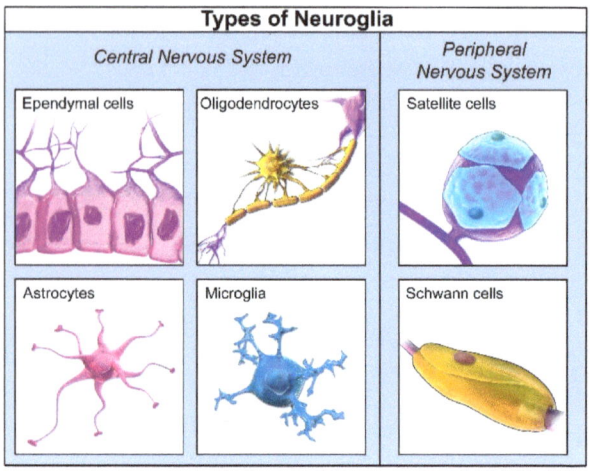

Figure 4-2 Types of glial cells

BY: Blausen.com staff (2014) "Medical gallery of Blausen Medical 2014," via wikipedia the free encyclopedia

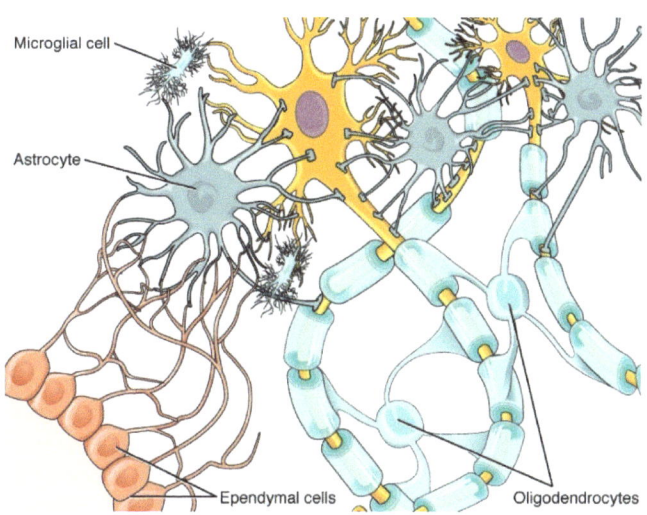

Figure 4-3 Glial cells of the CNN.

By OpenStax [(CC BY 4.0) (http://creativecommons.org/licenses/by/4.0)], via Wikimedia Commons.

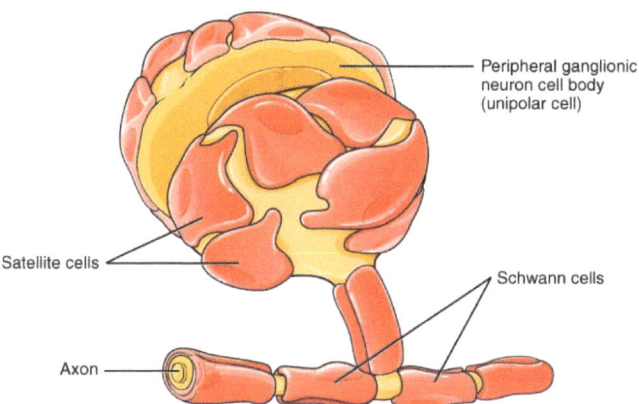

Figure 4-4 Glial cells of the PNS. By OpenStax [(CC BY 4.0), (http://creativecommons.org/licenses/by/4.0)], via Wikimedia Commons.

4.3 Oligodendrocytes

Have less branches than astrocytes and neurons. They warp their cell membrane around the neuron's axons to form a protecting coat (Schwann cells) that insulates the electrically conducting axons, which carry the action potentials, to avoid leakage and unwanted connections with other cells. See Figs. 4-2 and 4-3

4.4 Ependymal cells

They form the epithelial lining (ependymal) of the ventricular system of the brain and the central canal of the spinal cord, where they beat their little branches or cilia too impulse the cerebral-spinal fluid (CSF). See Figures 4-1, 4-2, 4-3 and 4-5. The ependymal cells participate in the creation and secretion of the CSF. Which fills all the ventricles located deep inside the brain and flows around the brain's outer rim. The CSF fluid also protects the spinal cord where 4/5 of the total amount of CSF is used. The CSF is produced by the **choroid plexus**, which consists of masses of tiny fingers, provided by ependymal cells, and blood capillaries. The choroid plexus is located in the lateral ventricles and in the fourth ventricle (inside the brain).

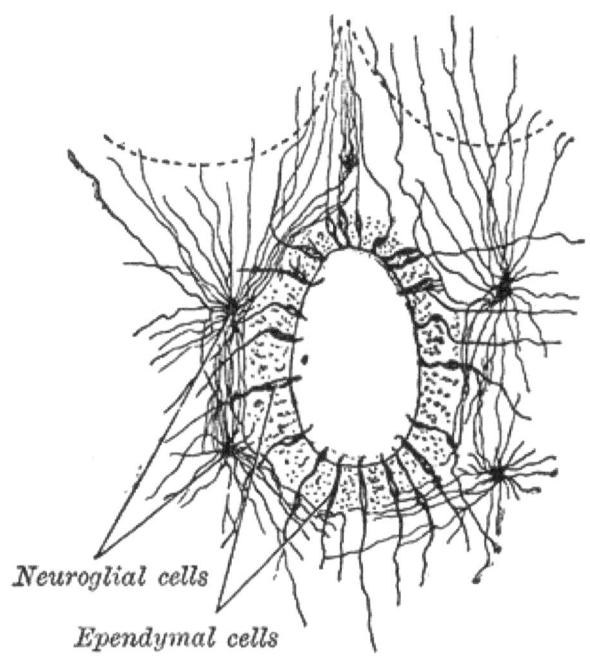

Figure 4-5 Illustration shows Ependymal and Neuroglial Cells. This image is in the public domain.

Author: Henry Vandyke Carter (1831-1897).

Chapter 5

Thinking About Thinking

5.1 Questions

1. How humans convert incoming information into a format that could be stored in our brain, and how do we actually store it?
2. How do we organize the incoming information and assign a storage location to it within our brain?
3. How do we compare and assign importance or priority to the incoming information?
4. How do we decide what could be discarded?
5. How do we recall the stored information, and how we decide which one is the pertinent one?
6. How do we decide which information should be discarded once used or which one should be memorized forever, never to be forgotten?
7. How the brain reaches conclusions and how it produces ideas, theories, and concepts?

These seven questions, (and for sure there are many more), are a big mystery and it will remain so for many years.

5.2 Humans thinking process

Our understanding of the human species thinking process is weighted by the restriction inherent in our reasoning process. The trail left by the following manifestation of our inherent restriction spans the entire field of scientific endeavors.

- The step-by-step procedure, which is the cornerstone of our scientific development, ties us to the prevailing knowledge.
- The mathematical entities available to express our rationalizations are very similar to each other.
- The step-by-step procedure is a fundamental part of the human species thinking process. Its mark is everywhere, but nowhere being it more obvious than in science.

This procedure prevents us from producing our best the first time around. In other words, we are not capable of producing from scratch the best we can. Humans need to use the prevailing knowledge to generate better and more complete knowledge. The step-by-step procedure is so ingrained in our mentality that it is hard for us to accept the possibility of any other way of creating. But a superior being with a less restricted mentality might produce the best it can without going through many cycles of confrontation between logic and experience.

Mathematics can be characterized as the operative treatment of symbols, where the meaning attached to a symbol is crucial to the power and elegance of the particular branch of mathematics that uses the symbol. Actually, the mathematical entities that we use to express our most powerful and pure thinking are very similar in the sense that they follow the same basic operational rules. This narrow spectrum of basic operational rules (which underlie all human symbolic rationalizations) is a very subtle but common restriction that affects our theories. For example, the following rules and laws of operations are common (some or all of them) to almost all the branches of mathematics, although there are **many** exceptions:
1. Subtraction is the inverse of addition.
2. Division is the inverse of multiplication
3. Division by zero is not defined
4. Addition and multiplication are commutative operations, that is, the order of the terms or factor does not alter the sum or the product.
5. Addition and multiplication are associative operations; that is, you can combine the terms or factors as you please.
6. Multiplication is distributive with respect to addition; you can multiply by each term one at a time, and then add.

5.3 Thinking restrictions

The mind produces theories, ideas, and concepts through reasoning and reasoning implicitly conveys restriction. Hence, man cannot make rationalizations without restriction. Bias and restriction are dissimilar concepts. Bias makes our thinking directional, limited, sluggish, and encroaches upon the full use of our mental capabilities. Restriction is inherent in the human species mental process and has an **organic origin.** It is an unknown function of the number of neurons and glial cells in the human brain and how they are organized and interconnected. Our restriction decreases the number of options available to the human **species** reasoning process when it is applied. It must have taken many millenniums after the first application of the human reasoning process to do the second successive application. From the very beginning, we used our reasoning (first application) process automatically to survive and to conduct our daily life. Sometime in the remote pass, our specie evolved and conducted the second successive application of our logic. That incorporated into our thinking process billions more of thinking components (neurons and glial cells), succinctly, we did a second application of our logic.

For a long time, human researchers have been looking for the "thinking molecule or organelle" that would explain how we think and memorize. They had found nothing, so the only thing left, to decipher the human reasoning process and how we memorize, is the patterns formed by countless millions of neurons and glial cells that are activated or illuminated during the thinking process. Let us call these giant groups of cells: thinking patterns or networks. Humans are the most intelligent animals on the planet, we can speak and clearly communicate with each other and present our reasoning using our spoken or written language. The human brain contains more than 200 billion neurons and a trillion glial cells and their interconnection patterns are the only thing left to explain our thinking process. When an action potential is fired by a neuron it reaches all its synapses with the same strength, and many of these synapses will in turn trigger additional action potentials in several thousand other neurons, and so on. It is an exponentially growing activation of neurons that proceed toward the intended targets and also must inform the CNS about the event that took place. No one knows where the propagation stops or how many neurons participated in it, but there must be a place in our brain that limit and direct all these activities. Regarding our thinking patterns, we have zero data, so the equation below is only a guess that must be confirmed before it could be accepted as valid.

$$N = k / R^n \quad (5.1)$$

N = Number of cells in the pattern
k = Constant during a logic application.
k is a function of n, for n = 1 is different than for an = 2
R = Restriction introduced by the application of the reasoning process
n = Order of restriction

$$k = N \cdot R^n \quad \text{k is in the range of } 10^6 \text{ to } 10^{10} \quad (5.2)$$

$$R^n = k / N \quad (5.3)$$
$$R = (k / N)^{1/n} \quad (5.4)$$
If n =1 $R = k / N$ (5.5)

Eq. (5.5) provides the restriction introduced by the first application of the reasoning process.

If n =2 $R = (k / N)^{1/2}$ To make a second application, the specie must be able to think with a value of R smaller than used in the first application.

The larger number of cells in the pattern the smaller R would be, the more interconnecting options the pattern would have. And the less restricted the thinking process would be. Every species has his own R. The order of restriction is the exponent of R, which in Eq. (5.1) is equal to **n**. Meaning the thinking process produce results with restriction of **order** n.

For a first application of a logic (thinking pattern), which is the regular case, n is equal to one. Meaning that when the target is not new, that it has been reached many times before, then the pattern produces results with restriction of order one (R^1). This would be always the case, except, for example, when humanoids / humans applied their logic successively (twice) to expand their understanding and obtain results which were completely new and very powerful. **Like going from sounds to spoken language.** This of course is a rare event, that required the evolution of the species (bigger head with more space for more neurons and glial cells) and for sure it must have taken many centuries to be completed. The size of the human head is limited by the size of the female womb and the duration of the gestation period. All in accordance with biped bone structure. Recent studies indicate that to accommodate the human brain development it was necessary to complete the gestation period outside the womb (external gestation). In fact, brain cells in the frontal lobes are still migrating at 6 months of age. It is a complicated subject, which is totally outside the subject of this book.

To clarify the concept of restriction, let us consider mathematics which is the **operative treatment** of the symbols created by the first application of our logic. Hence, mathematics is the result of a second application of our logic. For example: From Eqns. (5.4) and (5.5) we obtain:

$R = (k / N)^{1/n}$ (5.4)

If n =1 $R = k / N$ (5.5)   Restriction introduced by the first application of the human reasoning process.

The restriction of the mathematical symbols created during the **first application** of the human logic is given by Eq. (5.5). For instance, let us assume that $k = 4 \times 10^9$

and $N = 10^9$ then: **R = 4**. For the second application we use Eq. (5.4). Let us assume that k remains at the same value 4×10^9 and that the number of cells in the pattern also remains the same or 10^9, Substituting in Eq. (5.4) we obtain: **R = $4^{1/2}$ = 2** Restriction introduced by the second application of the human reasoning process.

The result of the example verifies that during the second application the species must think with a value of R smaller than in the first application.

Man is obviously the most advanced species on earth. Indeed, our logic is far superior to the logic of any animal. We are capable of abstract thinking, and we had conceived ideas, theories and concepts far beyond the reach of any other animal. *Compared to animals we are "something else."* Yet, due to man's evolutionary relationship with the other animals, the sensory organs (which determine the animal's experience of its world) of many animals are very similar to those of man. Furthermore, since both man and animals share the same planet, and hence the same stimuli, it is reasonable to conclude that the logic patterns of many advanced animal species closely related to man must be akin to man's logic. Though more restrictive, **larger R** in Eq. 5.4

IF IT IS ALIVE, IT THINKS! THEREFORE, ALL ANIMALS, CELLS AND ORGANELLES THINK, THERE IS NO OTHER WAY TO EXPLAIN THEIR PERFORMANCE.

Some examples of the **order of restriction** introduced by the human species logic in extending human knowledge are listed below:

Order of restriction of sounds with specific meaning.... 1
Order of restriction of spoken language........................ 2
Order of restriction of sound symbols............................ 1
Order of restriction of written language........................ 2
Order of restriction of any kind of symbols.................... 1

Order of restriction of mathematics................................ 2
Order of restriction of concepts... 1
Order of restriction of physical laws................................ 2

For sure, it must have taken a long time for the human species to apply his logic a second time. But once done, the other second applications took, for sure, much smaller time. For instance: To go from sounds to spoken language, it must have taken a very long time. But to go from sound symbols to written language, the time taken must have been much smaller. Once humans learned how to apply their thinking process a second time to expand the results obtained during the first application, they were effectively, *thinking with a smaller restriction (smaller R) and the number of neurons and glial cells utilized in their thinking patterns increased as required.* Once you have achieved the second application you must keep using it, you cannot go back, at will, and use the first application.

5.4 It is a humans' world

The human species already performed the second application of our thinking process. However, our abstract thinking is based on concepts that we created before the second logic application and on new concepts created as part of the second logic application. This is so because we are in the middle of the second application and our brain has all the necessary components and structures to implement and accomplish all that is possible with the second logic application. Although, we have accomplished a lot with the second application and reached very far. Sometimes we confront a problem that we cannot solve, regardless of how much we try. For instance, we cannot learn or explain how our brain works. It does not matter how much we desire to accomplish that goal, we cannot do it. Actually, we realize that we are very far from the target, and we are starting to suspect that we will never reach the target, that it is beyond human understanding. Something similar to what happen to dogs, which in the first application of their logic, they learned how to emit sounds with specific meaning. And they understand and obey our commands and you can see in their eyes that they want to talk, but they cannot do it. To accomplish that goal they would need to evolve and improve their brain, and then go into their second application, although with a larger R than the human R.

Chapter 6

Thinking Patterns

6.1 Introduction

Sensory organs contain sensory neurons adapted to respond to specific stimuli and conduct their nerve impulses to the brain. Sensory organs are very specific regarding the stimuli to which they respond, they act as frequency filters that allow perception of only a narrow range of frequencies. For instance, the rods and cones

within the eye respond to a precise frequency range of the incoming light waves and normally do not respond to x-rays, radio waves, or ultraviolet and infrared light. It is well documented how sensory neurons connect the sensory organs (vision, sound, odor, taste, and touch) with the central nervous system (brain, and the spinal cord). And we all have seen the specific locations of the brain that are stimulated, actually illuminated, when the human under test see objects, hear sounds, smell some odor, taste, or touch something. At any of these locations when a sensory pattern is activated, billions of cells, mainly neurons and glial cells start working. Some of these patterns are continuously activated even when the subject is sleeping.

Brain patterns are extremely complex not only because the extremely large number of components they contain. But because these components do not fit well our knowledge base. For instance, each brain pattern contains billions of ions, many of them with different charge values, different sizes and moving at different speeds, which are very slow when compared to free electrons and photons. In fact, the charge, sizes, and speeds (which are not constant) of the following ions, usually encountered within brain patterns, are all different K^+, Na^+, Ca^{++}, and Cl^-. The electric charges of these ions are multiple of the <u>electron</u> electrical charge, $e = -1.602 \times 10^{-19}$ coulombs. For example:

K^+: Potassium cation electrical charge $= - (-1.602 \times 10^{-19}) = 1 \times 1.602 \times 10^{-19}$ coulombs.

The present day knowledge about the brain patterns is almost zero. We know that each of these network contains billions of neurons, and even more of the many types of glial cells, and Schwann cells, and that blood capillaries provide blood to the pattern. The interactions between all these components is largely unknown. But what is completely unknown is *how we memorize information, and how we reason about it.*

In contrast, the analysis of electrical and electronic networks is based on electrons (not alive particle) and the analytical tool used are the Maxwell's equations. These equations are the "holy grail" of electrical engineering. But, for several reasons, is not practical to use them to decipher the thinking patterns. Besides the Maxwell equations do not contain photons, that we know are present, because during the activation of the thinking patterns, *they become illuminated.* These photons are part of the light reflected by the observed object.

The contemporary bias is to use quantum electrodynamics to explain the operation of the thinking patterns. Regardless of the tool used to study and analyze thinking patterns, *the fact is that there is a significant electric field present in any thinking pattern due to the very short distance of separation between electric charges.* The resultant electric field inside a thinking pattern is a function of its electrical charge distribution.

6.2 The electric and magnetic fields.

The concept of electric charge is well engraved in the human brain by centuries of observation of commonplace events. The theory of classical fields was developed back in the 19th century, when the interactions between the electric and magnetic fields was discovered by Gauss/Faraday and mathematically described by Maxwell in his famous differential equations. Latter expressed in vectorial calculus by Heaviside. Vector calculus formulas are full of the nabla (inverted capital delta) **vectorial operator**. The electromagnetic instantaneous power flow per unit transverse area is:

$$I = (1/\mu) \, E \times B \quad watt/m^2$$

Where
I is the instantaneous power flow vector in per unit
E is the electric field vector
B is the magnetic field vector
μ is the permeability of the medium
x means vector product

The vector intensity I is called the Poyntin vector, which is perpendicular to **B** and **E,** which are also perpendicular to each other. The vector **I** is in the direction of the electromagnetic wave propagation.

However, for calculating fields when the charge content of **a thinking pattern** is not homogeneous (different ions) and the charge distribution is asymmetric the use of differential equations provides the best chance of obtaining valid results if the thinking pattern is formed by a small number (never is) of particles.

Physic in general, and especially quantum physics, are built around elementary and virtual particles. Quantum electrodynamics is perhaps the most adaptable to decipher the thinking patterns, but it is far, very far, for what really is needed. The following knowledge has been part of our culture for many years:

- A changing magnetic field creates an electrical field, and the converse is also true.
- Electric and magnetic fields can exist in otherwise empty space and very remote from any material object. They travel at the speed of light in empty space.
- Electric and magnetic fields can coexist in the same space and constitute an electromagnetic field.
- Electromagnetic radiation, light included, consists of traveling electromagnetic fields. Which are setup and maintained by a self sustaining action in which one field creates the other. See Figure 6-1

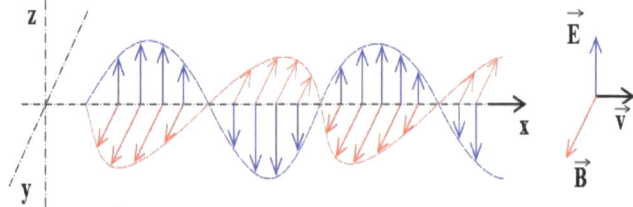

Figure 6-1 Electromagnetic wave illustration.

Licensed under the Creative Commons Attribution-Share Alike 3.0 Unported. (https://creativecommons.org/licenses/by-sa/3.0/deed.en) license.

6.3 Quantum electrodynamics

Based on the solid foundation described in 6.2, the concept of quantum fields was conceived and developed. Furthermore, the nature of the electromagnetic force is now described with great precision at the **elementary particle** level by the Quantum Electrodynamics (QED) theory. Full of the enthusiasm generated by the success of the QED theory in describing the electromagnetic force, we have reached the conclusion that the same pattern of reasoning must be valid for other forces in different spaces. The QED theory adopted the pattern set by Coulomb's law as the pattern to follow in describing the forces between elementary particles, **ions are not elementary particles**. The quantum electrodynamics theory, unlike the classic field theories, does not depend on the action at a distance concept; instead, the interaction between two particles is explained as the result of exchanging a virtual particle, which cannot be observed directly. The particle that conveys the electromagnetic force is a **virtual photon**, which, contrary to a real photon is unobservable. Furthermore, the absorption of a virtual photon does not transmute the absorbing particle into another kind of particle. A **real photon** is a particle of electromagnetic radiation that travels at the speed of light. It has energy, but does not have any rest mass or charge. Real photons are easily observable, as light is made of real photons. The electromagnetic force is explained in terms of **the constant exchange of virtual**

photons between the interacting particles. However, the exchanged of photons seems to violate the conservation laws of energy and momentum during the time interval between photon emission and photon absorption. The Quantum Theory accepts these violations provided that the excesses in energy and momentum are returned within the time and space constraints of the uncertainty principle. That is:

$\Delta t = h/\Delta E$ $\hspace{2em}$ $\Delta x = h/\Delta p$

Where

ΔE = Magnitude of the energy violation.
Δp = Magnitude of the momentum violation.
Δt = Time interval during which the violation is allow.
Δx = Uncertainty in position.

Elementary particles, and matter in general, have a dual nature. Some of their aspects could be explained using their wave properties; other aspects must be explained by their particle properties. However, if we insist on using only the particle model, then there are limitations on how precise we can be with this simplified model. Actually, the position and velocity of a particle cannot both be known precisely at the same time, and therefore the particle energy is uncertain during a small period of time (Δt). The Quantum Theory interprets the electromagnetic interaction between two particles as follows: The first particle emitted something that could not be seen or observed, and that something carried with it the missing energy and momentum and delivered it to second particle. This something that could not be observed is called a virtual photon. To make the whole transaction legal, physicists imposed time and space limits within which this shuffle is tolerated; outside these limits the conservation laws are strictly enforced. The introduction of virtual particles

into the scheme of things affected some very basic concepts; actually anything can happen in the "twilight zone" of the Webner Heisenberg uncertainty principle, like:
- Virtual photons can spontaneously germinate out of empty space, survive the time allowed by the uncertainty principle, and then disappear.
- Electrically charged virtual particles can also be created in empty space, provided that the charge conservation law is not violated. Therefore, they are created and destroyed in pairs of particles and antiparticles. For instance, an electron-positron pair can spontaneously sprout from a photon, virtual or real. Actually, the pair would be quickly annihilated and converted back into a photon.

The symbolic expression of Coulomb law is:

$F = k (Q_1 Q_2) / d^2$ where k is a proportionality constant. This law only applies when the size of the charges is very much smaller than the distance separating them. Actually, **Coulomb law was written assuming point charges, which are infinitely small.** The force F acts along the line joining the two point charges (Q_1 and Q_2). If the two charges have the same sign, the force is repulsive, it would be attractive if the charges are of different signs. The Coulomb equation can be transformed to express the strength of the electric field interaction independently of the of the separation distance and the units used to express this separation, as follows:

The electric charge in particles are quantized. That is, any charged particle, with the exception of quarks, have an electric charge that is an integral multiple of the proton charge (no intermediate values.) Therefore, the interaction between two protons has the minimum possible value of the electromagnetic interaction. So it is convenient to define the electric charge of a proton as the unit of electric charge. Evaluating the Coulomb law for $Q_1 = Q_2 = 1$ we obtained the factor k/Hz, a dimensionless number which provides an absolute measure of the strength of the electromagnetic interaction. It is called the **coupling constant**. Symbolically:

$Fd^2 = k(Q_1Q_2)$ $\qquad$ $Fd^2/hc = k(Q_1Q_2)/hc$
if $Q_1 = Q_2 = 1$ $\qquad$ $Fd^2/hc = k/hc$

Electromagnetic coupling constant = k/hc dimensionless number = $1/137 = 0.0073$. According to the QED theory, the coupling constant of the electromagnetic interaction is not constant, but actually increases at very close range, this is when the separation of the interacting charged particles is smaller than 10^{-12} centimeters.

6.4 Vision and the human eyes

Below I provide a very brief and elementary description of the human eye and its operation. The reader should understand that the subject matter is very complex and that I left out a lot of information. Figs. 6-2 to 6-7 support the description.

Here is what happens when we see something. The light reflected, **the stimulus in this case**, by the observed object enters the human eye through the cornea and *penetrates the pupil, and then go through the crystalline lens, which controlled by the ciliary muscles focuses the light beam on the photoreceptor cells located in the retina where the light is converted into an electrical signal which is delivered by the optic nerves to a specific sensory pattern located in the brain.* How the brain converts the electrical signals into the image that we see is totally unknown. Although we know where in the brain the signals go. See Fig. 6-7.

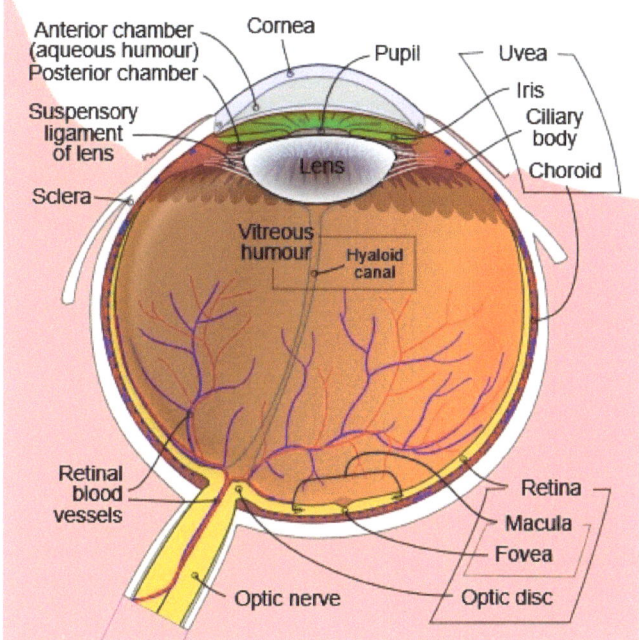

Figure 6-2 Cross section of the human eye
By Rhcastilhos [Public domain], via Wikimedia Commons.

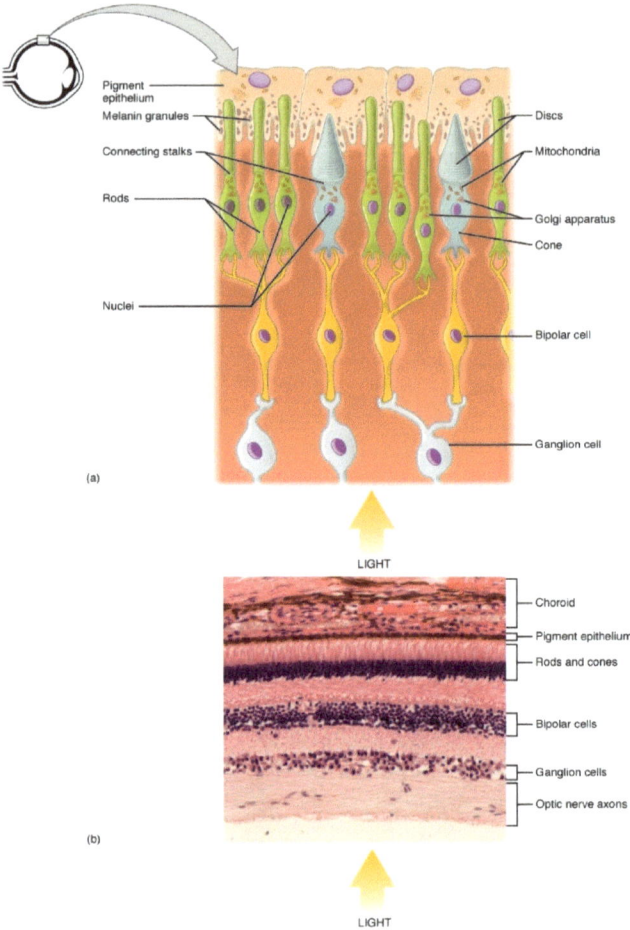

Figure 6-3 Retina's structure. By creative Commons Attribution 3.0 unported license.

"*http://creativecommons.org/licenses/by/3.0/deed.en_US*"

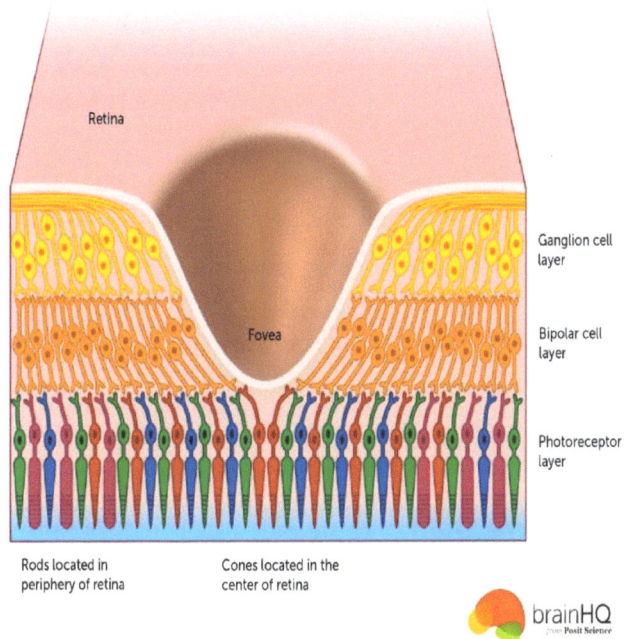

Figure 6-4 Illustration shows the distribution of cones and rods in the fovea area. **Original from Posit Science.**

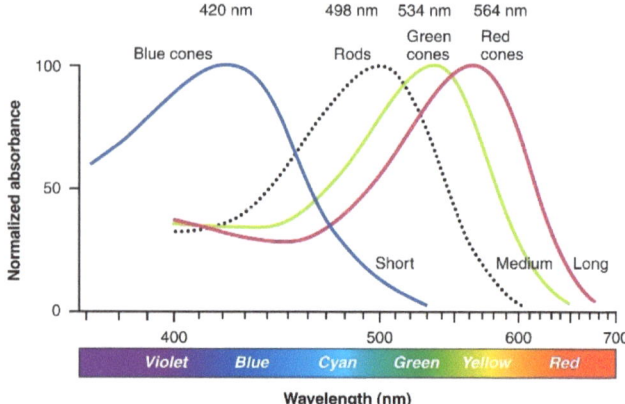

Figure 6-5 Response of cones to light spectrum.
By OpenStax College[(CC BY 3.0)
(http://creativecommons.org/licenses/by/3.0)], via Wikimedia Commons.

6.5 The retina Is a membrane that consists of many layers. See Figs. 6-3 and 6-4.
1. The nerve fiber layer which is the outermost layer and is the first one crossed by the reflected light, <u>actually everything in the macula could be considered as simultaneous illuminated, by the reflected light.</u> The nerve fiber layer is formed by nerve cells and blood capillaries.
2. The ganglion cell layer
3. The inner plexiform layer
4. The Inner nucleous layer
5. The outer plexiform layer
6. The outer nucleous layer
7. The photoreceptors (Rod and Cones) layer.

8. The retinal pigmented epithelium that contains melanin to reduce light scattering inside the eyeball.

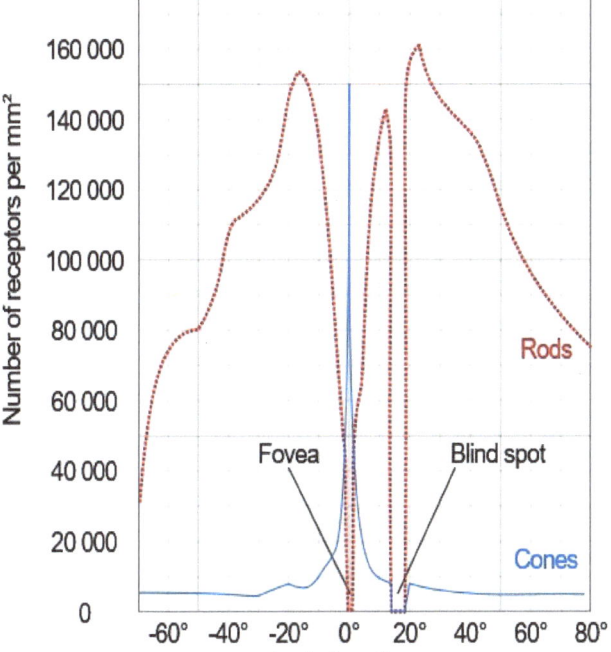

Figure 6-6 Population of photoreceptors in the most sensitive part of the retina. Licensed under the Creative Commons Attribution-Share Alike 3.0 Unported license. **GNU Free Documentation License**, Version 1.2

In the retina the incoming reflected light is converted into DC electrical signals, which is send to the brain via the nerves in the nerve fiber layer. It is a common mistake to call these electrical signals "Action Potentials." All action potentials have the same wave shape and therefore they cannot transmit information. Besides action potentials are very slow because they depend on chemical synapsis. The visual perception must be transmitted, exclusively, by electrical synapsis. The retina is populated by many millions of five types of neurons: photoreceptors, bipolar, ganglions, horizontal, and amacrine cells. Actually, the visual perception is basically transmitted from the eye to the brain by a compact arrangement of four types of components, all of them located in the retina: *photoreceptors (rods and cones,) bipolar cells, ganglion cells and optical nerve.* See Figs. 6-3 and 6-4.

The perception start when the lens in the eye focuses the reflected light into the photoreceptors in the Macula/Fovea area, located on the rear portion of the retina, and where resides the most sensitive area of the retina. See Figs 6-4. The photoreceptor neurons could be of two different shapes: **rods and cones.** Rods are bigger than cones and most of them populate the area of the macula at the left and right of the fovea. See Figs. 6-4 and 6-6. There are about 120 million rods in the retina and they are very sensitive to light, so they could be excited by dim light and therefore they are good for night vision. There are about 6 million cones in the retina. And most of the them are located in the fovea, at the center of the macula area; there are not rods in the fovea. See Fig. 6-6. Cones respond very well to high intensity light and are the ones we use for tasks that require high acuity perception. Besides, cones are the photoreceptors that provide us with color vision. In fact, there are three different types of **cones** accordingly of how they respond to the frequency of the reflected light: red, green, and blue. The reader should keep in mind that the frequency spectrum of the reflected light could contain all the visible colors or only one of them. The cone outer segments, formed by a stack of decreasing diameter disk-like pieces, are covered with a photopigment material, which is of a different type for each cone-color, that respond very well to a specific color frequency of the reflected light, meaning that some cones generate a V_R, DC voltage when illuminated with red light, others cones generates a V_G, DC voltage when illuminated with green light, and the remaining cones generate a V_B, DC voltage when illuminated with blue light. **Actually, any specific cone type responds to a range of frequencies or wavelengths**, for instance a red cones respond to light within the wavelength range of 400 to 700 nanometers, but the peak of the response occurs at a wavelength of 564 nanometers. However, at that wavelength the green cones are also responding, although with less intensity. Actually, combining the outputs of the three types of cones, we could see the entire gamma of colors, more or less.

The electromagnetic field propagation (reflected light) ends at the retina. Actually, in the fovea is where the electrical and magnetic fields contained in the incoming light are separated. **The electromagnetic field of the reflected light mimics, exactly and instantaneously the shape, size, and color of the object that reflected the light. There is not another plausible explanation.**

I **believe** the vision, sensation is developed as follows: The output voltage (in the range of two to four volts) generated by the cones and rods is delivered to a **specific sensory pattern** in the brain. Riding on top of the DC output voltage generated by the photopigments, there is a small signal, in the millivolt range, that contains the information brought-in by the electromagnetic field of the reflected light. So, the electrical signal delivered to the brain contains all the necessary information which allows us to see in color the observed object. There is no theoretical reason to consider that vision-images are only transmitted electrically or chemically. It could well be that the electromagnetic wave signals propagate inside the brain, where the extracellular space is fluid-like, and the path length is only five or six inches. Furthermore, the highly mobile Glial cells could play a role in the electromagnetic wave propagation inside the brain. The visual cortex is the largest pattern in the human brain. It is located at the rear of the brain above the <u>cerebellum</u>. See Fig. 6-7.

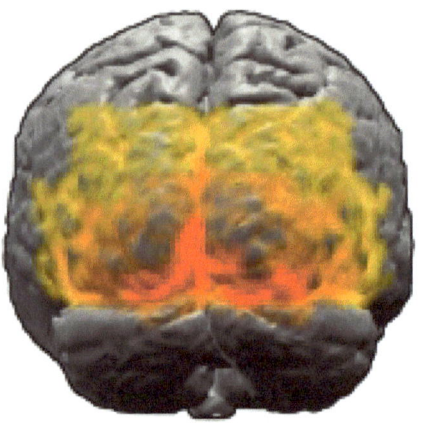

Figure 6-7 Brain area activated when observing an object. By The original uploader was Washington irving at English Wikipedia [GFDL (http://www.gnu.org/copyleft/fdl.html) or CC-BY-SA-3.0 (http://creativecommons.org/licenses/by-sa/3.0/)], via Wikimedia Commons

6.6 Sensory patterns

Let us **assume** that the electrical signal transmitted from the retina to the sensory-pattern in the brain mimics, instantaneously, the information contained in the incoming stimulus (the reflected light) and which is the image of the object that reflected the light. Furthermore, the **shape** of the equipotential surfaces in the electric field created by the electrical signal transmitted to the brain is determined by the information contained in the light reflected by the observed object. So, the information contained in the stimulus is directly correlated to the shape of the equipotential surfaces in the sensory pattern. We don't know yet, how the brain can convert, instantaneously, the shape of the equipotential surfaces into a visual image. It might be significant that the glial cells prefer to be on the equipotential surfaces of the electrical field, because in this way they conserve energy when they move. A large area of the brain participates in the vision sensation, larger that the area taken by any other sense. Part of this area is shown in Fig. 6-7.

I hope that the reader realize that the patterns associated with the human senses would be the simpler ones, if you could compare them to the memorizing and rationalization patterns.

6.7 Alzheimer's brain disease

The present consensus is that Alzheimer's is produced by amyloid-beta plaques located around and close to the brain cells, neurons and glial cells. Or by tangles of misfolded Tau proteins formed in the neuron's tracks. These plaques and tangles could increase the number of dead cells beyond the brain removal capacity of dead cells. Scientis are now studying the dynamic of this problem at the molecular and cellular levels. In fact, the main fields of research for curing Alzheimer's are plaques, tangles and dead cell removal.

Plaques are composed of small protein fragments or peptides called amyloid-beta (Aβ). Actually, A-beta is a fragment of a protein called Amyloid-beta Precursor Protein or APP. The APP molecule consist of a chain of amino acids that live anchored to the neuron (or to any human cell) membrane. The APP molecule works one way while complete and in a different way after broken in pieces. When it is complete it contributes to the growth and repair of the neuron's membrane. And it is also a leading participant in many other neural processes. However, after breaking in pieces, two of these pieces create the infamous A-beta peptide.

Actually, the APP molecule could be cut in two different ways by two different sets of enzymes. The set that creates the infamous A-beta peptide is the **beta-secretase and the gamma-secretase set.** See Fig. 6-8. The APP is a long and multifunction protein that consists of four pieces interconnected by flexible linkers. The beta secretase cut high the APP molecule liberating the top fragment which is soluble in the watery environment of the extracellular fluid. The gamma secretase cuts the chain inside the neuron's membrane, leaving a fragment attached to the plasma membrane and liberating the amyloid-beta (Aβ42, 42 amino acids) peptide, which has adhesive properties, into the fluid environment of the extracellular space. Many of the A-beta peptides liberated by the surrounding neurons cling to each other, forming long and flexible filaments. An entire collection of these filaments interlace one with another, forming a chaotic looking, disk-like (or ball-like) structure, called The **Amyloid Beta plaque** (A-beta). A-beta plaques accumulate between neurons and because they are toxic to neurons they induce their inflammation, which call the attention of the immune system phagocytes and microglia, which in due course will swallow or break-eat the disabled neuron. Besides, the Aβ42 interferes with the ionic and molecular traffic across the neuron's plasma membrane. Which is another factor that contributes to the premature death of neurons and brain destruction. See Fig. 6-9. In contrast, the tau protein, mostly lives inside the neuron's axon (none in dendrites) and plays a role in the formation and stability of parallel strands, these strands are called **tracks.**

These tracks are made from beta-amyloid fragments and heavy phosphorylated Tau proteins. The tracks are part of the neuron cytoskeleton, which transport neuron's synthesized ingredients from the neuron body to the presynaptic terminals, at the end of the axon, and to all other neuron's dendrites. **The straight and well organized tracks could collapse into a tangle-looking mess called tangles. Tangles are made of hyperphosphorylated and misfolded tau proteins.** Actually, the tau proteins when hyperphosphorylated and **misfolded** could form very insoluble **tangles** of paired (helical and straight) filaments.

We know the following about Alzheimer's:
- Is not an infection disease
- It is a very slow developing disease

And we could **guess** that is produced by the following:
1. The lack of a specific nutrient; or perhaps is due to the repetitive ingestion of a specific nutrient or eating too much of it, or due to the involuntary absorption of a chemical ingredient.
2. The slow removal of dead cells in the brain.
3. Harmful ingredients (cells, molecules, ions, atoms of heavy metals, etc.) that might come by way of the blood or the cerebral-spinal fluid entering the brain.

4. By overwhelming our skull with damaging electromagnetic radiation during dental and medical appointments.
5. In any of the many cell's patterns, the number of inactive cells increases with age. This is so because the information contained or the function performed by some specific cell becomes obsolete, not required anymore. These cells might decide that it's time to claim its independence and migrate outside the pattern. In doing so they could be flushed away by the cerebral-spinal fluid or the blood, which will transform them (digested) into something else. This process would reduce the size and density of the brain, and therefore its capacity to control the human body.

Of course, drinking alcohol or smoking marijuana is a very efficient way of destroying your brain. However, this subject is beyond the scope of this book.

Regarding the involuntary absorption of chemical ingredients or elements, the obvious path is the digesting system. However, for cell-damaging ingredients to get into the brain via the digesting system the process is well known, but complicated and long. Conversely, absorption of brain-cell damaging ingredients or elements through the tissue lining the mouth cavity is an improbable but uncomplicated way of reaching and harming neurons and glial cells.

I believe, that the most important thing to avoid the Alzheimer's disease is to maintain the death rate of neurons and glial cells below the removal capabilities of glial cells, phagocytes, or any other cell that help with the removal of dead brain cells. Hence, It would be a step in the right direction to stimulate the immune system which would increase the available phagocytes.

Things that I do:
- While at home, I don't use toilet paper (It contains a lot of chemicals) anymore. Instead, I use a gadget installed in the toilet, that very quickly and completely, clean and refresh the anus with a jet of fresh water. If you desire, you could adjust the temperature of the water, it does a perfect job! No more staining your underwear with disgusting compressed excrement. You could buy the gadget online or in the local store.

- After brushing my teeth I rinse my mouse several times, until the water is clear.
- I shake really well, my underwear before I used.
- I avoid ingesting artificial products, like artificial sugar.
- I eat lots of parsley and fruits because they contain phytochemicals, which some of them, I believe (big guess) are beta-secretase and gamma-secretase **inhibitors.**

Phytochemicals are protective chemicals that plants (fruit and vegetables) use to fight diseases. Although, phytochemicals are not an essential nutrient for humans, it has been established that some of them can also protect humans, among them lycopene (tomatoes), flavonoids (fruits), isoflavones (soybean) and lutein (corn).

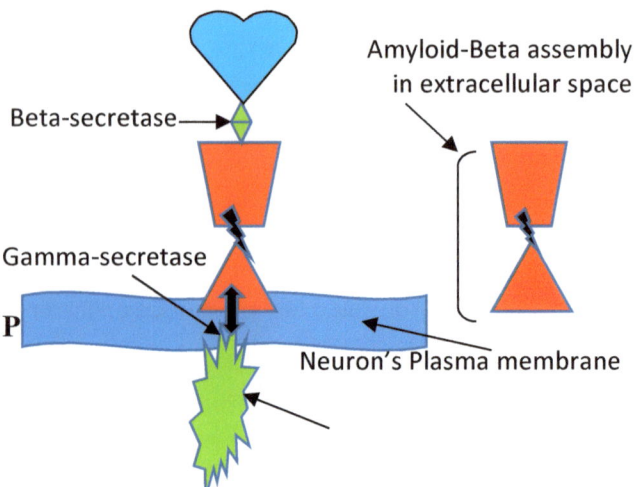

Figure 6-8 Illustration of Amyloid Beta creation.

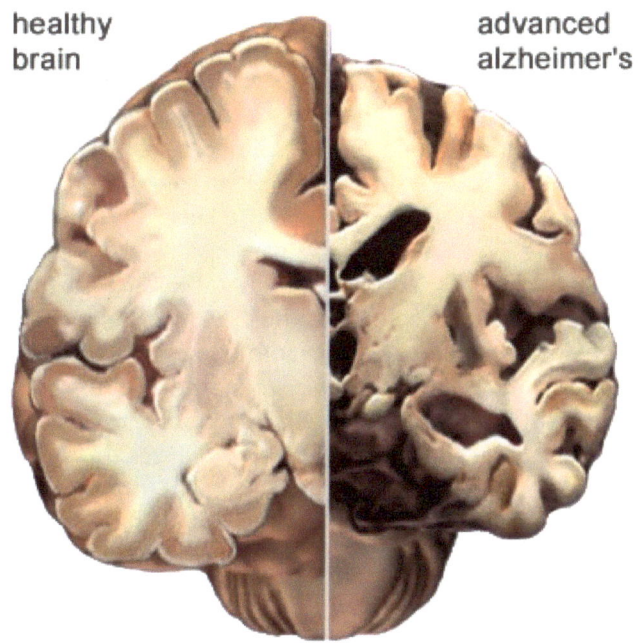

Figue 6-9 Brain comparison. Jannis Productions. Stacy Jannis (CC BY 3.0).

6.8 Neural Networks and Artificial Intelligence

At the present time artificial neural networks are built around artificial neurons, specifically, Sigmoid Neurons which behind this fancy name are nothing more than NAND gates. Initially, the technology was based on Perceptron NAND gates. The output of Perceptron's could only be zero (0) or one (1), the voltage value of a (1), depends on the rating of the power supply energizing the network. In contrast the output of Sigmoid Neurons could be zero, any intermediate value between zero and one, or one. In fact, to design and built a smart neural network, we need artificial neurons capable of delivering a **linear output**, such that a small change in the weight assigned to one of the artificial neuron's inputs or to the bias assigned to the artificial neuron itself, produces a small (proportional) change in the output. In fact, Sigmoid Neurons are actually trainable because they can deliver a linear output. They could be trained, using learning algorithms, to automatically tune the output, according to the application, and according to the existing experience, to an acceptable value. Furthermore, external stimuli (like in the human brain) should trigger the auto-tuning without the operator or the network programmer approval, it just happens! This human like characteristic moves neural networks in the direction of robots.

Smart machines are machines that execute a set of instructions to accomplish a specific task. To do a different task, it requires another set of instructions and to properly set the machine to accomplish the new task. These are the smart machines that most car-assembly plants use. This type of machine performs heavy work and they require an external supply of electrical power, usually provided by input electrical cables connected to the plant electrical system. These machines cannot move outside the small working area assigned to them. In fact, they are limited by the length of the power cables.

The following fictional narrative would help to clarify what a robot should be capable of doing.

*DATE: Summer of 2077, 2:15 am **(night time)***

Place: Shipping yard of a local Receiving and Delivering Company near a metropolitan city in the USA

Robot 1 gets close to robot 2 and ask: "What are you doing?"

Unloading tomato boxes. "How many boxes to go?" "Let's see… 48"

"I need you in Lot 4 to help me with the handling of some radioactive containers."

"Sorry, but first, I need to finish with these boxes. The tomatoes are almost ripe and they would need to be discarded after four or five days."

"These are orders from the General Manager! You go ahead and tell him you cannot do it."

"Yes, sir, I will do it. After I get a quick charge. It would take, at least 75 minutes."

"Shit… You are impossible… why you didn't tell me that before…."

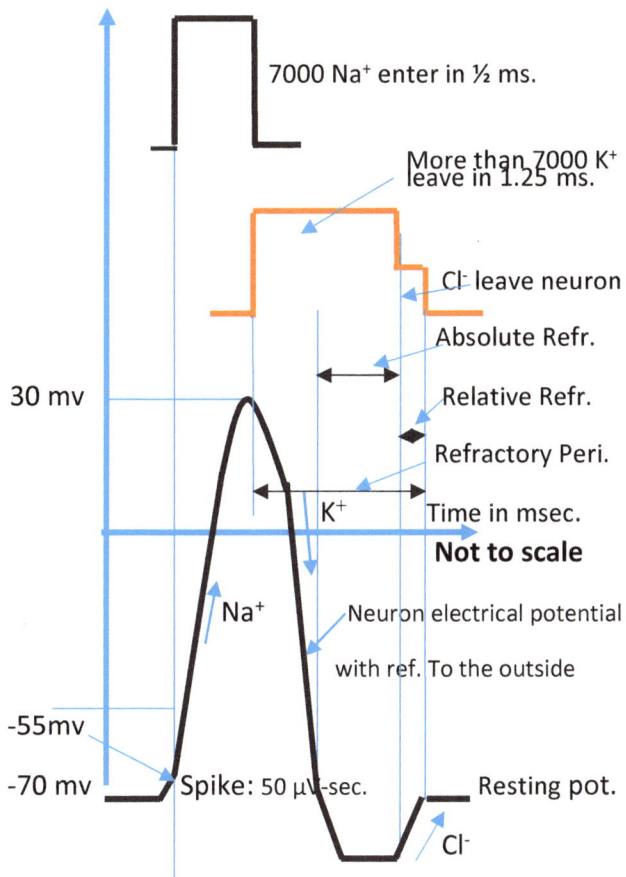

Appendix 1: Action Potential Illustration

www.ingramcontent.com/pod-product-compliance
Lightning Source LLC
Chambersburg PA
CBHW041101180526
45172CB00001B/50